The Changing Face of Medical Education

The Changing Face of Medical Education

Edited by

PENELOPE CAVENAGH
Director of Research and Enterprise
University Campus Suffolk

SAM J LEINSTER
Professor of Medical Education
School of Medicine, Health Policy and Practice
University of East Anglia

and

SUSAN MILES
Research Associate in Medical Education
University of East Anglia

Foreword by
Professor Shirley Pearce
Vice Chancellor
Loughborough University

Radcliffe Publishing
Oxford • New York

Radcliffe Publishing Ltd
18 Marcham Road
Abingdon
Oxon OX14 1AA
United Kingdom

www.radcliffe-oxford.com
Electronic catalogue and worldwide online ordering facility.

British Library Cataloguing in Publication Data

A catalogue record for this book is available from the British Library.

ISBN-13: 978 184619 457 3

The paper used for the text pages of this book is FSC® certified. FSC (The Forest Stewardship Council®) is an international network to promote responsible management of the world's forests.

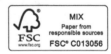

Typeset by Pindar NZ, Auckland, New Zealand
Printed and bound by TJI Digital, Padstow, Cornwall, UK

Contents

Foreword

The education of our healthcare professionals is one of the most important challenges for higher education. Society needs us to prepare doctors who are able to solve complex problems, understand research, implement technological advances, gain patients' trust, operate in multidisciplinary and multi-agency teams and, on a continuous basis, access and integrate knowledge from many different sources. To do all this effectively requires a tremendous range of skills and knowledge as well as an ability to reflect on one's own personal qualities and style.

To prepare students for the world in which they must work we need to understand these complex tasks and also understand how people learn to deliver excellence in meeting them. We need also to understand the best way to help students reflect on their own development and make the right career choices. Medicine is a wonderful profession in this respect as there are so many branches within which one can practice and which demand different kinds of skills and expertise.

In setting up the new medical school at UEA we recognised this challenge and set out to develop a method of teaching and learning that put the student and their learning needs at the centre of the curriculum. The content of the learning and teaching methods used to facilitate that learning were carefully developed from an evidence base that was grounded in educational theory. The team setting up the new school looked at innovations in educational practice across the world and sought the advice of experts with experience of delivering innovation that had been shown to be effective. The commitment was to deliver a learning programme that was developed on the basis of what has been shown to work rather than what tradition dictates. The results of this and some of the developments that have emerged from those early days are outlined in this book.

Some basic principles guided the delivery of the new medical school:

> All innovation should be based on evidence of its efficacy.
> Accordingly, theory and practice should be integrated from the outset of training so that the framework of knowledge that guides doctors' decision making is developed around the real-life problems that doctors see in practice.
> The reality that many medical students gain employment in primary care rather than hospitals should be reflected in the curriculum by increasing the opportunities for primary care experience and providing clinical experience in primary care from the beginning.
> Recognising the multidimensional nature of health and illness and so teaching the full range of psychosocial, physiological, anatomical and biochemical factors that influence health in an integrated way.
> Recognition that healthcare is delivered by multidisciplinary teams. This brings breadth of knowledge and expertise. It can also bring inter-professional rivalries and problems of communication. The best way to prevent this is to educate different health professions together. Not by sharing lectures but by sharing consideration of clinical problems and drawing on the growing evidence on inter-professional learning.

These requirements were built into the new curriculum and this book shows the outcome a few years on. The team developing the new medical school had the privilege of working from a 'clean slate' and I am proud to have been part of that original team. The credit for delivery, however, goes to the team of people who delivered our vision. Many of these people are authors to the ensuing chapters and I have the greatest respect for what they have done.

Medicine changes all the time. Our priorities for intervention change. We develop new treatments, new methods of working, new methods of illness prevention. We must make sure that our educational programmes for doctors reflect the sophistication of these changes and that we do not become ossified in what we teach and how we teach it. Introducing evidence-based change in learning methods is relatively easy to deliver from scratch. Much more difficult is to ensure that new evidence for improved learning is regularly introduced into an established curriculum.

This is a challenge to a new medical school as much as it is to a well-established school and so I am pleased to see serious review and reflection built into the UEA Medical School's development. It is great to see the openness with which the authors of this book have approached the task and this summary of progress and issues raised so far will, I am sure, stimulate all of us to review what we do and incorporate examples of great practice.

My warmest congratulations to all who have been part of the delivery of the changes in medical education that we have seen, not just at UEA but also right across the country. I am convinced that the needs of the patient and the health of the nation will have benefited from these innovations, and the commitment to continue to question and improve our methods of teaching and learning that this book promotes.

Professor Shirley Pearce
Vice Chancellor, Loughborough University
November 2010

About the editors

Dr Penelope Cavenagh
Director of Research and Enterprise
University Campus Suffolk

Professor Sam J Leinster
Professor of Medical Education
School of Medicine, Health Policy and Practice
University of East Anglia

Dr Susan Miles
Research Associate in Medical Education
University of East Anglia

List of contributors

Dr Lesley Bowker
Clinical Skills Director and Honorary Senior Lecturer
University of East Anglia

Dr Laura Bowater
Lecturer in Medical Education
University of East Anglia

Dr Sandra Gibson
Lecturer in Medical Education
University of East Anglia

Professor Christopher Hand
Deputy Director MB/BS Programme
University of East Anglia

Professor Amanda Howe
Professor of Primary Care
University of East Anglia

Dr Barbara A Jennings
Senior Lecturer in Molecular Medicine
University of East Anglia

Dr Alexia Papageorgiou
Lecturer in Consultation Skills
University of East Anglia

Dr Gill M Price
Lecturer in Medical Statistics
University of East Anglia

Dr Louise Swift
Medical Statistician
University of East Anglia

Dr Richard Young
Practice Development Tutor, MB/BS Programme
University of East Anglia

CHAPTER 1

The history of change in the UK

Sam J Leinster

Medical education is widely regarded as a very conservative part of a conservative profession but in the early 1990s change swept through UK medical schools. Medical school curricula, which had been relatively homogenous, became diverse in terms of teaching methods and content, although all are required to meet the learning outcomes set by the General Medical Council in *Tomorrow's Doctors*. At the same time medical education began to develop as a distinct specialty with its own units and departments. Universities began to appoint professors of medical education, some of whom were clinicians while others were educationalists or psychologists. In parallel with these changes Government policy led to an increase of medical student numbers by 40%. Some of this increase was met by enlarging class sizes in existing medical courses; some was met by the creation of shortened graduate entry courses alongside the traditional courses in established medical schools; some was met by the creation of new medical schools.[1] For those involved there has been a perception of unprecedented rate and extent of change almost amounting to a revolution.

Formal regulation of medical education in the UK began with the Medical Act of 1858 which established the General Council for Medical Education and Registration and gave it authority to determine what constituted adequate education for a registered medical practitioner. Prior to that date the regulation of the medical profession was a local matter with a degree of rivalry existing between the various Universities and corporations that were entitled to award a licence to practise within their territory. The training for licensure differed among the various bodies. The Universities of Oxford, Cambridge and London awarded a Licentiate, a Bachelors degree and a Doctorate in Medicine. Study within the University was focused on Classics and Mathematics. Medical studies were usually pursued elsewhere although the examinations took place in the University. The Graduates of Oxford and Cambridge claimed the right to practise anywhere in England except for London where the practice of medicine was controlled by the Royal College of Physicians. This right was disputed by the Apothecaries Hall in London who claimed the right to limit general practice in London to Licentiates of their corporation. Licensure was given following a 5-year apprenticeship.[2] The practice of surgery was controlled by the Royal College of Surgeons who tried to keep surgery distinct from the practice of medicine. The College's diploma was viewed unfavourably by some senior members of the medical profession on the grounds that its examination was too restricted and therefore the diploma was too easily obtained. Although diplomates were only tested on their knowledge of surgery they went on to practise in other fields of medicine. This was actually illegal but the law was not enforced.[3]

Similar arrangements were in place in Scotland. The College of Surgeons of Edinburgh was originally incorporated in 1505 and granted a Royal Charter by James IV in 1506. Its original seal of cause states:

> . . . that no manner of person occupy or practise any points of our said craft of surgery . . . unless he be worthy and expert in all points belonging to the said craft, diligently and expertly examined and admitted by the Masters of the said craft and that he know Anatomy and the nature and complexion of every member of the human body . . . for every man ocht to know the nature and substance of everything that he works or else he is negligent.[4]

Its authority was, however, limited to controlling the practice of surgery in Edinburgh and eight counties in the south-east of Scotland. In contrast, the Royal College of Physicians of Edinburgh had authority only within the old walled city.

Whatever the shortcomings of these institutions the real scandal was the large number of poorly educated and unlicensed practitioners who provided medical care for the greater proportion of the population.

The pressure for change had been evident for many years. In 1800, the Provincial Medical and Surgical Association published a monograph on the principles on which the reform of the medical professions should be based. They emphasised the need for a sound knowledge of basic science combined with adequate clinical training. By 1826 no real change had taken place but a new University was about to be created in London and it was going to have a medical school. There was no shortage of advice to the Council of the University on what form that medical education should take. In *Thoughts on Medical Education* 'Medicus'[5] set out his suggestions for admissions criteria (Latin, Greek and mathematics); the duration of studies (2 years); and the outline of the curriculum. He suggested three phases – introductory, progressive and clinical. The introductory phase was to be the natural sciences – natural history, systematic botany and descriptive anatomy. The progressive phase comprised natural philosophy (physics), chemistry, phytology, physiology and moral philosophy. During this phase the student would be expected to attend the anatomy room for 2 hours daily to undertake dissection. The clinical phase was to cover Materia Medica and Pharmacy; Pathology and the Practice of Medicine; Surgery; Obstetrical Surgery and Medicine; Medical Jurisprudence; and Medical Ethics. During this phase the student was expected to attend clinical lectures in various hospitals, continue dissection in the anatomy department and carry out post-mortems as often as possible. The emphasis on a balance between basic science, clinical studies and the humanities has a curiously modern ring.

Following its establishment the General Medical Council (GMC) (as it came to be known) maintained a close scrutiny on the nature and content of medical education in the UK. From as early as 1863 concerns were expressed that the medical curriculum was overloaded and did not allow the student time for self-education.[6] This charge was to be repeated at regular intervals until 1993. At the same time new disciplines were added to the course and new material was added to old disciplines as medical knowledge grew. The difficulties of remedying this situation were increased by the Medical Act of 1886 which required that the graduate should possess 'the knowledge and skill requisite for the efficient practice of medicine, surgery and midwifery'. As postgraduate education was not required it followed that nothing could be omitted from the undergraduate curriculum. This legal requirement was not removed until the revision of the Medical Act in 1978 and 1983.

While attempts were being made to reform medical education in the UK, the situation in the USA remained chaotic. There were excellent institutions providing sound scientific and clinical education but there were many private medical schools awarding 'qualifications' after minimal periods of study. Other practitioners were receiving their training from unregulated apprenticeships. The public had no way of distinguishing properly trained physicians among the practitioners on offer. Andrew Carnegie, the philanthropist, was so concerned that he commissioned Abraham Flexner, a well-known educationalist, to enquire into the state of medical education. Flexner published his report in 1910[7] and then visited Europe to report on the situation on the Continent and in the UK. He published his report on this visit in 1912. These two documents were to exert a major influence on medical education throughout the 20th century.[8]

Flexner identified the need for a sound education in science as a basis for medical education. He also emphasised the need for formal clinical instruction. In his review of Europe he praised the German teaching of the basic sciences while holding up the British system of clinical instruction as an example. The system of medical education that developed became the universal pattern throughout the world. A period of 'pre-clinical' scientific studies was followed by a period of formal 'clinical' education usually known as *clerkships* in North America and *firms* in the UK. The relative lengths of the phases varied and the overall duration of the course was between 4 and 6 years.

The introduction of the Flexner curriculum coincided with the beginnings of the rapid expansion in medical knowledge which has gathered pace with time. As early as 1918 the great physiologist Ernest Starling highlighted the need for basic medical training to include aspects of public and community health. He went on to acknowledge that although there were complaints of the curriculum being overloaded, no one could say that any of the introduced subjects were unimportant.[9] He expressed concern that despite the load of factual knowledge the students were still poorly prepared for practice. His main complaint was that the graduates lacked breadth of culture, understanding of scientific principles and a facility for acquiring new ideas, all of which are necessary if medicine is to develop. Despite such erudite concern the content of the curriculum continued to grow while the overall time available remained static.

In 1944, the Ministry of Health for England and the Department of Health for Scotland asked Sir George Goodenough to undertake a review of medical education in order to determine how best to prepare doctors for the proposed National Health Service.[10] The committee focused on the process of medical education, making recommendations with regard to the structure, funding and staffing of medical schools. They did, however, comment on the need for curricular reform with attention needing to be paid to social medicine, child health and mental health if the newly qualified doctors were going to be fit to serve in a National Health Service which would be as much about health promotion and preventive health as the treatment of individuals with disease. An important recommendation was the creation of a compulsory *pre-registration year* following graduation in recognition that it is impossible to learn all that is needed for the safe practice of medicine in its varied branches in 5 years. It was to be almost another 10 years before this suggestion was adopted in law and 14 years before it became operational. The concept that the undergraduate curriculum could not be expected to provide sufficient training for the immediate unsupervised practice of medicine, was reinforced by the Todd Report in 1968 which also reaffirmed the need for significant curriculum reform.[11]

Sir George Pickering in 1978 re-iterated the need for curricular reform.[12] He suggested that the principal purpose of undergraduate medical education should be to train the student's mind to enable him to reach a judgement. This necessitated developing attitudes such as curiosity and awareness as well as cognitive skills such as collecting and assessing evidence.[13]

The medical students whom he interviewed in the preparation of his report stressed the importance of teaching teachers how to teach; a concept that he endorsed. He highlighted good practice in some medical schools that had removed the control of the curriculum from departmental heads and vested it in curriculum committees. These schools tended to have a measure of integration between subjects and an increased emphasis on community-based medicine. However, many schools continued to follow the traditional curriculum.

The GMC urged curriculum change in its recommendations in 1957, 1967 and 1978. Some minor changes of curriculum configuration occurred but the fundamental problem was not addressed.[14] The authors of *Tomorrow's Doctors* in 1993 could complain that there was still a drive towards completeness in the curriculum which arose from the reluctance of departments to surrender any of their teaching time.[15]

The burden of factual knowledge required in order to pass the examinations became so great that students were forced into superficial learning approaches, memorising swathes of knowledge with little opportunity to develop understanding of the subjects or habits of critical enquiry and thought. As a result, they were often unable to apply their knowledge to a specific patient in a clinical setting.

As medical knowledge grew and new sciences developed, the emphasis in academic medicine shifted from teaching to research. Status, kudos and career progression became contingent on success in research that was defined in terms of grants obtained and papers published. Teaching was not recognised as a discipline with its own set of knowledge and skills.

This combination of factors led to increasing disillusionment among medical students. A number of authors identified the problem that British medical schools were attracting high-calibre students who became disillusioned as a result of the teaching they received.[16]

TOMORROW'S DOCTORS (1993)
Against this background the GMC produced a series of recommendations for basic medical education in 1993 entitled *Tomorrow's Doctors*. A major part of the recommendations was that factual overload should be reduced by the defining of a *core curriculum* which every student should be required to undertake. This was to occupy no more than two-thirds of the available time. The other third would be allotted to *Special Study Modules* whose main purpose would be the development of intellectual skills such as curiosity and critical thinking. The underlying objectives for medical education set out in the document were similar to those in previous reports, as the authors themselves acknowledged. It is therefore reasonable to ask why the 1993 recommendations produced such major changes in both the content and the delivery of the curriculum in many medical schools in the UK.

EXTERNAL DRIVERS FOR CHANGE

While the Education Committee of the GMC was debating the nature and contents of their recommendations, the King's Fund published a report on a national consensus inquiry into medical education.[17] Coincident with the publication of *Tomorrow's Doctors* there was a series of influential articles by Stella Lowry in the *British Medical Journal* under the general theme of 'What's wrong with medical education in Britain?'.[18] The series covered the major aspects of the course from student selection to curriculum design and delivery. It provided a useful synopsis of the views of a growing band of educationalists and psychologists who had an interest in medical education and suggested solutions from successful medical schools outside of the UK. Because it was published in the *BMJ* rather than a specialist education journal it reached a wide audience of influential decision makers within the medical profession.

INTERNAL DRIVERS FOR CHANGE

Within the medical schools there was an increasing awareness that students were dissatisfied. The extent of this dissatisfaction was reflected in a successful BBC series broadcast in 1992, *Doctors to Be*, in which a considerable number of the students interviewed expressed disillusionment with their choice of career. The negative view that students had of medical school was reflected in falling application rates to all medical schools.

THE ROLE OF THE CHIEF MEDICAL OFFICER

An important factor in the implementation of changes in medical education in 1993 was the decision of the then Chief Medical Officer for England, Sir Kenneth Calman, to fund curriculum facilitators in every medical school. This resulted in an influx of educators from a variety of backgrounds who brought a fresh approach to the challenge of teaching medicine. Prior to this point it was unusual for people involved in the teaching of medicine to have any form of qualification in education. The ensuing dialogue between the biomedical specialists and the educational specialists proved to be fruitful. New approaches to teaching, learning and curriculum development became widespread. While there is no way to quantify the impact of appointing the curriculum facilitators, they appear to have been an important factor in the changes that took place. They were often a catalyst for the establishment of medical education units or departments within the schools. When the initial Department of Health funding ran out the majority of medical schools maintained the posts from other resources.

THE FUNCTION OF MEDICAL EDUCATION UNITS

Traditionally, the curriculum in medical schools was the responsibility of the individual departments. The central administration of the medical school was responsible for determining which departments it would support and how much time for teaching was allotted to each department. The GMC requirements that graduates should be competent in medicine, surgery and midwifery shaped the finals examinations but the actual content and nature of the teaching was left to the departmental heads. The GMC call for greater integration of subjects in teaching led many schools to set up centralised curriculum committees which were responsible for determining the form and content of the curriculum. These committees were in existence before *Tomorrow's Doctors* but their influence was often limited. Departments continued to wield power because of the perception that they were the subject experts and therefore best placed to determine what should be taught. The existence of centralised committees made it easier for medical education units to influence the curriculum as they were usually regarded as the natural source of expert educational advice for the committees. Since the members of the medical education units were involved in the national associations where there was active debate on modern, theory-based approaches to education, these ideas influenced the deliberations of the committees.

THE RISE OF MEDICAL EDUCATION AS A DISCIPLINE

It is generally accepted that all doctors have a duty to teach the rising generation of practitioners. This laudable obligation has been distorted into the belief that all doctors are automatically capable of teaching without further training.

In 1957, a group of doctors who were interested in medical education came together to form the Association for the Study of Medical Education. The Association is a learned society that provides a forum for individuals interested in medical education to develop their theoretical and practical understanding of the subject.

Its original objectives were:

➤ To exchange information about medical education
➤ To organise meetings on topics concerning medical education
➤ To maintain a bureau where information about medical education is collected, stored and made available
➤ To encourage, promote and conduct research into matters concerned with medical education.[19]

From an early stage it welcomed non-medical members with relevant expertise and interests in medical education and encouraged innovation and research. In 1966, it published a journal, *The British Journal of Medical Education* (now known as *Medical Education*) that has gone on to become the leading international journal in the field. In 1972, the Association for Medical Education in Europe was founded. The two associations overlap in membership and officers. Between them they have been responsible for transforming medical education from an activity of enthusiastic amateurs to an increasingly professional discipline. The meetings organised by the associations are an important factor in the dissemination of good practice and provide forums where new approaches to education could be debated and evaluated. The journals *Medical Education* and *Medical Teacher* (published by the Association of Medical Education in Europe) have not only played a role in educating the teachers but, with their function as learned journals, have encouraged the development and spread of research into medical education which has been an important factor in the self-identification of the discipline.

PROFESSIONAL MEDICAL EDUCATORS

The literature provides evidence that there have always been doctors who have been interested in teaching and have seen engaging with medical students as a crucial part of their own professional persona. Nevertheless, teaching has usually been seen as a natural talent rather than a skill to be acquired, and medical students have been tolerated as a necessary evil rather than recognised as an essential part of the continued development of the profession. Academics were identified by their clinical or scientific disciplines and made their reputations within that discipline. Academic promotion came as a result of distinction within the discipline.

The Centre for Medical Education in Dundee[20] was founded in 1975 and began running training courses for medical educators. These eventually grew into a Postgraduate Certificate in Medical Education and then a Masters in Medical Education. Other centres followed suit and it is now commonplace for medical schools to run Masters programmes in medical education.

Within the broader field of Higher Education there was growing concern about the quality of teaching. As a result a Register of Professional Teachers has been established. Initially, this was run by the Institute for Teaching and Learning in Higher Education – it is now run by the Higher Education Academy.[21]

The past 15 years has seen the appointment of academics who have medical education as their designated discipline. In the early days many of these individuals were already established as academics within their own disciplines. The criteria for appointment varied from medical school to medical school but the common reason was engagement in curriculum design and reform. In 1990, there was no Professor of Medical Education with an interest in undergraduate education in the UK. There are now over 20, with an increasing cohort of senior lecturers and lecturers supporting them. Increasingly, junior doctors are opting for training in medical education as part of their professional development and expecting a career where progression will depend on their educational expertise and activity.

WHAT OF THE FUTURE?

It seems likely that medical education will become even more professionalised to the point where it will be recognised as a separate specialty within medicine. There are dangers inherent in this. One of the strengths of medical education, particularly in the clinical components, is that it has been delivered by individuals who are still active in clinical practice. As a result, there has been coherence between developments in practice and the students' learning. The students become caught up in the teachers' concerns for their patients as well as their enthusiasm for their discipline. Medical educators who are not practising clinicians run the risk of becoming outdated in their medical knowledge and blunted in their response to patients' changing needs. On the other hand, clinicians who have no expertise in education will not achieve the maximum advantage for students from the teaching sessions they undertake.

The best quality of patient care now occurs when a range of specialists and sub-specialists work together as a team. In a similar way, future medical education will be most effective if the medical education specialist is part of a team working closely with clinicians to decide the best approaches to delivering teaching in an increasingly pressured environment.

REFERENCES

1 Howe A, Campion P, Searle J et al. New perspectives: approaches to medical education at four new UK medical schools. BMJ. 2004; **329**: 327–31.

2 'Medicus'. Thoughts on Medical Education and a Plan for Its Improvement. London: Longman, Rees, Orme, Brown and Greene; 1827. pp. 5–6.

3 'Emeritus'. A Letter on Medical Registration and the Condition of the Medical Corporations. London: Jackson; 1852.

4 Royal College of Surgeons of Edinburgh. History of the College. www.rcsed.ac.uk/site/345/default.aspx (accessed 9.5.2010)

5 'Medicus', ibid. pp. 16–18.

6 Cited in Tomorrow's Doctors. London: General Medical Council; 1993.

7 Flexner A. Medical Education in the United States and Canada: a report to the Carnegie Foundation for the Advancement of Teaching. Reproduced in Bulletin of the World Health Organization. 2002; **80**(7): 594–602.

8 Cooke M, Irby DM, Sullivan W et al. American Medical Education 100 years after the Flexner Report. New Engl J Med. 2006; **355**: 1339–44.

9 Starling EH. Medical Education in England: the overloaded curriculum and the incubus of the examination system. BMJ. 1918; **2**: 258–9.

10 Editorial. The training of doctors: report by the Goodenough Committee. BMJ. 1944; **July 22**: 121–3.

11 Royal Commission on Medical Education (1965–8). Report to Parliament. Cmnd 3569. London: Her Majesty's Stationary Office; 1968.

12 Pickering G. The Quest for Excellence in Medical Education. Oxford: Oxford University Press; 1978.

13 Ibid. p. 37.

14 Bloom SW. Structure and ideology in medical education: an analysis of resistance to change. J Health Soc Behav. 1988; **29**: 294–306.

15 General Medical Council. Tomorrow's Doctors. London: GMC; 1993. para 17.

16 Fraser RC. Undergraduate Medical Education: present state and future needs. *BMJ.* 1991; **303**: 41–3.

17 Towle A. *Critical Thinking: the future of undergraduate medical education.* London: King's Fund; 1991.

18 Lowry S. What's wrong with medical education in Britain? *BMJ.* 1992; **305**: 1277–80.

19 www.asme.org.uk/images/History_of_ASME_book.pdf (accessed 10.5.2010)

20 www.dundee.ac.uk/meded/frames/home.html (accessed 10.5.2010)

21 www.heacademy.ac.uk/ourwork/supportingindividuals/professionalrecognition (accessed 10.5.2010)

CHAPTER 2

The effects of traditional medical education

Penelope Cavenagh

The traditional process of becoming a doctor and the accompanying sociali-sation effect has been deemed to be so powerful that it has been likened by a senior doctor to 'getting your hand caught in a meat grinder'[1] which gradu-ally grinds you into a uniform package until you 'pop out as a doctor'.[1]

The personal cost of 'popping out' as a doctor after this intense training period appears to have been very high for some medical students. A review of stress, coping and health during medical training[2] concluded that time at medical school resulted in psychosocial deterioration of medical students, and this was attributed to the stress of the educational process. The system of medical education was criticised by the General Medical Council (GMC) as early as 1863 in terms of the overcrowding of the curriculum and lack of time for self-directed learning.[3]

Despite these early criticisms, the 'status quo' of medical education remained for more than a century, providing a rich and fertile ground for numerous research studies carried out by educationalists, sociologists, psy-chologists and doctors. Investigations have mainly been along the lines of the immediate and long-term effects of this socialisation and educational process on medical students, the way they learn, their development as doc-tors and their psychosocial well-being.

This chapter summarises the key issues which have emerged from empirical studies on the effects of traditional medical education on students and which have contributed to the rationale for the revision of the medical curriculum with goals and objectives set out by the GMC in *Tomorrow's Doctors*.[3]

Traditional medical education consisted essentially of a two-year preclinical lecture-based course, followed by three years of clinical training that took place mainly in hospital settings. These two phases have also been described in terms of the 'pre-cynical' and 'cynical' years,[4] referring to evidence that shows the increasing cynicism of medical students as they progress during their medical training.[5,6]

The pre-clinical course drew on a spectrum of scientific disciplines, with information imparted didactically in a formal lecture theatre style. This formal setting is more conducive to passive styles of learning, rather than active acquisition of information.[7]

The relationship between basic science and clinical departments has been described in terms of 'mutual condescension' and 'strained tolerance'[8] and the curriculum as being 'driven by factual content and dominated by departmental rivalries over core knowledge'.[9]

This division between the pre-clinical and clinical aspects of medical training is believed to have inhibited the connection between 'scientific questioning' and 'clinical practice'[9] – and could ultimately 'impede innovative solutions to health concerns'.[9]

The quantity of factual content to be learned, incessant examinations and assessments, and the consequential effects on medical students is a recurrent theme in the literature.[10,11]

> They [medical students] will be expected to study more and learn more facts than is at all reasonable. There will be repeated assessments and examinations and they will need to discover strategies to enable them to cope with this load.[12]

In order to cope with the huge volume of facts in a context where assessments essentially involve the recall of factual knowledge, evidence suggests that students may develop coping strategies in terms of matching their learning styles to the outcomes required of them.[13] However, the strategies adopted may not be in the best interests of the educational process and present a short-term rather than lifelong approach to learning.

Research on approaches to learning in Sweden[13] show that students can be adaptable in their use of either a surface or deep approach to learning. The surface approach is a technique whereby students use rote learning to remember the key facts and ideas that they will have to recall in examinations. This is in contrast to the deep approach that involves the desire to genuinely understand and integrate issues, rather than rely upon factual recall.[14]

A study of learning behaviour in two medical schools[15] found that students showed little inclination to learn anything other than what they were told to. The analytic rather than independent learning styles adopted were unlikely to predispose the medical students to become effective lifelong learners. The conclusion from a review paper[14] on the implications of learning styles for medical schools suggests that students' perceptions of the medical course:

> may encourage surface or highly strategic approaches to learning neither of which is likely to produce a graduate with a well-developed capacity for critical thinking, problem-solving or self-directed learning.[16]

Survival tactics in terms of styles of learning have perhaps been adopted by medical students in the pursuit of avoiding failure and passing examinations at medical school, but despite this coping strategy there is agreement[17] that the vast quantity of information to absorb in traditional medical education has been a source of significant stress to medical students.

Key recommendations for the new curriculum[3] include a substantial reduction in the amount of factual information and a curriculum that engenders the capacity for lifelong learning and assessment strategies that reflect these learning styles. A call was also made for the end of the division between the pre-clinical and clinical parts of the medical course, as this split was deemed to be a critical factor in curriculum overload.

However, the inescapable reality is that training to become a doctor necessitates a lot of learning and it may be this alone or the context of an 'uncaring educational environment'[17] that has made medical education a distressing experience for some.[10,18,19]

> Concern has been expressed about the alienation and emotional blunting
> induced by the teaching style and competitive environment in which learn-
> ing takes place.[20]

Traditionally, medical students have been isolated physically by being
housed in a medical school, often away from the main university campus,
but also isolated mentally by the sheer bulk of work and relentless examinations. Medical schools have been likened to asylums or prisons where the
academic demands

> will ultimately result in professional cognitive membership of the institution
> of which they are an inmate – a passage and membership that may exclude
> the lay world just as surely as asylum walls.[21]

It could be hypothesised that medical students became more heavily
socialised into their future 'doctor' roles than other professionals because
of their constant interaction with the medical world and relative isolation
from society.

The environment in which medical education has taken place has been
depicted as 'authoritarian' and 'dehumanizing'.[22] Medical students' experiences of 'pervasive perceived mistreatment'[2] appear to be widespread and
have perhaps induced the 'emotional blunting'[20] described.

Negative emotions have been aroused in medical students, particularly
in their relationships with consultants, and incidents of public humiliation
have been frequently described by recipients of this unwanted behaviour.[19]
Feelings of dehumanisation in medical students have been partly attributed
to the lack of care or support given to them in a supposed caring profession.[23] An erosion of compassion witnessed in some doctors[24] may be
attributed to this 'personal deprivation' experienced as students.[23]

> It is ironic that in training for a profession which offers vast opportunities
> for self-actualization, individuals should undergo so many personal depriva-
> tions. One suspects that these deprivations eventually color the behavior of
> physicians in their practice of medicine.[25]

A basic derision of illness, particularly psychological, may account for these
behaviours towards students. Some doctors lack awareness or will not admit

to their own psychological problems and it seems that they would not want to be viewed by their colleagues in the same way that they see some of their patients.[26]

Recommendations for the new curriculum[3] include the desire to foster in a doctor the need to combine both scientific and humanitarian approaches to professional care, which would necessitate compassion and concern for patients' dignity.

Evidence suggests that, despite the introduction of the new curriculum, these desired attributes may not have been embedded effectively in medical students. The importance of compassion to medical students as a quality essential to being a doctor was found to decline in a longitudinal study in two medical schools.[27] Communication skills and compassion were the two most frequently mentioned qualities on entry to medical school, but had declined in frequency of response by the final year. This applied to medical students on both the old and new curriculum. This outcome could be explained in terms of previous research in Canada[28] that found that a large number of students on both the old and new curriculum (and particularly in their clinical years) did not consider their teachers to be adequate role models for how they should relate to patients. The response was based on the observed lack of compassion and caring shown to both students and patients:

> The lack of role models is likely to threaten the acquisition and nurturing of humanistic skills and attitudes by future physicians. It may also lead students to believe that these skills do not constitute an essential and integral part of their role as physician.[29]

Issues of 'psychoanalytic transference' have been raised as a possible explanation for some of the difficult and stressful relationships between junior doctors and their seniors. A longitudinal study[30] that examined the aetiology of job stress in terms of the contribution of the organisation vis-à-vis the individual followed-up junior doctors from when they were medical students. Junior doctors (assessed as students) who described their fathers' relationships to them as 'relatively more powerful, strict, intolerant and unsupportive' also reported higher levels of stress caused by senior doctors. Teaching hospital senior doctors provoked more stress in junior doctors than non-teaching hospital senior doctors.

The author hypothesised that teaching hospital senior doctors may be 'more critical and unsupportive' than their non-teaching hospital counterparts, and thus perhaps more at risk of inducing 'transference issues' in those doctors who have less favourable relationships with their fathers. The findings of this research are pertinent to the nature/nurture debate, what type of person chooses to study medicine and their reasons why. It may be that there is a certain personality type who is attracted to the profession.

Some research in the late 1960s, openly acknowledged as rudimentary,[31] showed that first-year medical students were more likely to display authoritarian tendencies than peer groups in the arts faculty. The study added weight to the author's suspicions that medical students and doctors seemed to possess a certain cluster of personality characteristics remarkably similar to those of the 'authoritarian personality'.[32] These characteristics are described as a bias towards

> subjects with a substantial body of precise information; a generally tough-minded attitude towards people, with a lack of sensitivity to their feelings; an identification with the powerful groups in society, with a consequent mistrust of minority groups.[33]

Whether these characteristics are innate or the result of medical training is questionable.[31]

Very few studies exist concerning medical students' choice of medicine as a career, and those that do are mainly retrospective and may be subject to recall bias. However, one prospective study of first-year medical students in Norway[34] found that person-orientated motives were the most important reasons for choosing medicine as a career for both men and women, with women scoring higher than men in this index. Women were nearly as motivated as men for status, security and interest in natural sciences.

These findings were replicated in a longitudinal study[27] following-up medical students on both the old and new curriculum in two medical schools in the UK. 'Working with people' and 'scientific interest' were the two most frequent responses for choosing medicine as a career given on entry and exit for both types of curriculum in each medical school. However, regardless of the type of curriculum, medical students emerged from medical school less happy and less committed to their choice of career than they were on entry.

The socialisation process at traditional medical schools can be summarised as a complex interaction of variables,[2] including those of personality. However, it seems reasonable from the evidence to speculate that the process may account for high levels of stress and psychological morbidity in some undergraduate medical students,[19,10] and perhaps for the prevalence of psychological and addictive behaviours in some qualified doctors.[18]

The big question for medical educators, the medical profession, their regulating bodies and indeed all patients is how successful has the new curriculum been in reducing stress levels in medical students, creating a learning environment conducive to active lifelong learning and producing well-rounded and competent doctors with humanitarian attitudes towards their patients?

Indications to date are generally positive about the ameliorating effects of the new curriculum. The end of the division between pre-clinical and clinical years, the introduction of problem-based learning (PBL), earlier contact with patients and greater interaction with teachers all seem to have conspired to give a better experience at medical school.

Research[35,36] suggests that the reformed medical curriculum fosters more supportive attitudes from teaching staff towards students than the traditional curriculum. This, in turn, may reduce negativity and hence stress in students, which should enhance the learning experience.[35]

A Norwegian study[35] showed that the positive effects of the reformed curriculum survived the entire medical student experience and this was attributed to greater personal contact with teachers. However, in a Canadian study, the effect was only shortlived[28] and although the PBL curriculum resulted in better relationships between faculty and students in the pre-clinical years than the traditional curriculum, the difference was not sustained in the clinical years.

Early positive interactions with medical teachers do appear to be an important factor in students' satisfaction with their learning environment, and it is tempting to conclude that the positive effects of the redesigned curriculum on reformed medical education programmes will only be sustainable if some of the traditional role models in clinical settings change and adapt some of their behaviours accordingly.

Further 'positive' effects from the use of the new curriculum have been demonstrated in terms of learning styles. Using the traditional programme, the amount of information to be absorbed produces a tendency towards superficial or surface patterns of learning which are not considered to be effective strategies for developing independent or lifelong learning. Recent research[37] has compared learning patterns from students following the traditional, innovative (PBL) and integrated curricula (PBL and traditional). Medical students on the innovative curriculum demonstrated deeper learning styles and more self-regulation of learning content than students on the other curricula. They also showed a stronger vocational commitment.

These findings were confirmed in another study[38] where medical students' experiences of their curriculum and the development of their learning strategies were compared within both a PBL environment and a traditional setting. The PBL students demonstrated a greater propensity for self-regulated learning, which had the additional benefit of preparing them for transition through medical school and ultimately for lifelong learning.

Tomorrow's Doctors[3] succinctly summarises the extrinsic and intrinsic factors that have catalysed modifications to the traditional medical curriculum and informed guidance on structure, styles of delivery and learning in a revised curriculum. External influences for change have included evolving and progressive technologies, advances in medical knowledge and the consequential emerging moral and ethical issues, an ageing and multiracial population, and consideration of the health of the population as a whole.

This chapter has focused on factors intrinsic to the curriculum that have contributed to change and on the context and culture in which traditional medical education has been delivered. Empirical studies discussed in this chapter have tended to highlight the negative impact of the traditional medical curriculum, particularly in terms of the stress induced by the intensity and assessment of this learning package and the portrayal of the unsupportive environment in which it is delivered.

Perhaps the ultimate cost of this style of education may be measured in terms of the high rates of psychological morbidity reported in medical students and doctors, and the personal cost to patients who may be on the receiving end of reduced levels of compassion and empathy from their doctors.

Recent studies have indicated favourable comparisons between the revised and traditional curricula, particularly in terms of learning styles and support given during this learning period. But we must trust that the baby has not been thrown out with the bathwater with the new curriculum and that some perceived negatives have not been misconstrued. For example, it has been questioned[17] whether compassion can be awakened in would-be doctors if it is not already an inherent aspect of their personality, and indeed whether perhaps 'clinical duty' should be the main drive for treating illness rather than compassion. The stress of medical education is also challenged in terms of varying individual responses to stress and the need to cater for those 'who thrive on the atmosphere of challenge'[17] and looming deadlines. Furthermore, a healthy dose of cynicism is suggested for perhaps improving the efficacy of treatment in particular cases.

We all have differing expectations of the medical profession and individual preferences for how we wish to be treated. Rather like pilots and flying, surely our first concern must be that doctors are clinically competent, practise evidence-based medicine and are safe practitioners.

We would all hope that any medical education, through its teaching, learning and assessment strategies, would ensure that these primary outcomes are achieved. If this can be delivered within the context of a supportive educational and clinical environment, where medical students are nurtured in a way that feeds their own humanity and encourages their thirst for learning and knowledge, then with effective recruitment strategies a revised curriculum should achieve the aspirations outlined for *Tomorrow's Doctors*.

REFERENCES

1 Coombs RH. *Mastering Medicine*. Chicago, IL: Free Press; 1978. p. 3.

2 Wolf TM. Stress, coping and health: enhancing well-being during medical school. *Med Educ*. 1994; **28**: 8–17.

3 General Medical Council. *Tomorrow's Doctors (recommendations on undergraduate medical education)*. London: GMC; 1993.

4 Becker HS, Geer B. The fate of idealism in medical school. *Am Sociol Rev*. 1958; **23**: 50–6.

5 Eron LD. Effect of medical education on medical students' attitudes. *J Med Educ*. 1955; **10**: 559–66.

6 Wolf TM, Balson PM, Faucett JM *et al*. A retrospective study of attitude change during medical education. *Med Educ*. 1989; **23**: 19–23.

7 Nandi PL, Chan JNF, Chan CPK *et al*. Undergraduate medical education: comparison of problem-based learning and conventional teaching. *Hong Kong Med J*. 2000; **6**(3): 301–6.

8 Coombs, op. cit. p. 46.

9 MacLeod SM, McCullough HN. Social science education as a component of medical training. *Soc Sci Med.* 1994; **39**(9): 1367–73.

10 Guthrie EA, Black D, Shaw CM *et al.* Embarking upon a medical career: psychological morbidity in first-year medical students. *Med Educ.* 1995; **29**: 337–41.

11 Radcliffe C, Lester H. Perceived stress during undergraduate medical training: a qualitative study. *Med Educ.* 2003; **37**: 32–8.

12 Bennet G. *The Wound and the Doctor.* London: Secker and Warburg; 1987. p. 97.

13 Marton F, Säljö R. On qualitative differences in learning – II – Outcome as a function of the learner's conception of the task. *Br J Edu Psychol.* 1976; **46**: 115–27.

14 Newble DI, Entwistle NJ. Learning styles and approaches: implications for medical education. *Med Educ.* 1986; **20**: 162–75.

15 Vu N, Galofré A. How medical students learn. *J Med Educ.* 1983; **58**: 601–10.

16 Newble, Entwistle, op. cit. p. 174.

17 Deary IJ. Need medical education be stressful? *Med Educ.* 1994; **28**: 55–7.

18 Firth-Cozens J. Emotional distress in junior house officers. *BMJ.* 1987; **295**: 533–6.

19 Firth J. Levels and sources of stress in medical students. *BMJ.* 1986; **292**: 1177–80.

20 Buckley EG. Basic medical education in transition. *Med Educ.* 1993; **27**: 113.

21 Sinclair S. *Making Doctors.* Oxford: Berg; 1997. p. 113.

22 Knight JA. *Doctor-To-Be. Coping with the trials and triumphs of medical school.* New York: Appleton-Century-Crofte; 1981.

23 Edwards MT, Zimet CN. Problems and concerns among medical students – 1975. *J Med Educ.* 1976; **51**: 619–25.

24 Weatherall D. The inhumanity of medicine. *Br J Med.* 1994; **309**: 1671–2.

25 Edwards, Zimet, op. cit. p. 625.

26 Sinclair, op. cit.

27 Cavenagh P. Medical students' beliefs and attitudes towards the doctor's role: is management seen as an integral part of this role? *Clin Management.* 2002; **11**: 199–220.

28 Maheux B, Beaudoin C, Berkson L *et al.* Medical faculty as humanistic physicians and teachers: the perceptions of students at innovative and traditional medical schools. *Med Educ.* 2000; **34**: 630–4.

29 Maheux *et al.*, op. cit. p. 634.

30 Firth-Cozens J. The role of early family experiences in the perception of organizational stress: fusing clinical and organizational perspectives. *J Occup Organiz Psychol.* 1992; **65**: 61–75.

31 Bennet, op. cit.

32 Adorno TW. *The Authoritarian Personality.* New York: Harper and Row; 1969.

33 Bennet, op. cit. p. 89.

34 Vaglum P, Wiers-Jenssen J, Ekeberg Ø. Motivation for medical school, the relation-ship to gender and speciality preferences in a nationwide sample. *Med Educ*. 1999; **33**: 236–42.

35 Gude T, Hjortdahl P, Anvik T *et al*. Does change from a traditional to a new medical curriculum reduce negative attitudes among students? A quasi-experimental study. *Med Teach*. 2005; **27**(8): 737–9.

36 Kiessling C, Schubert B, Scheffner D *et al*. First-year medical students' perceptions of stress and support: a comparison between reformed and traditional track criteria. *Med Educ*. 2004; **38**: 504–9.

37 Van Der Veken J, Valcke M, Muijtjens A *et al*. The potential of the inventory of learning styles to study students' learning patterns in three types of medical curricula. *Med Teach*. 2008; **30**: 863–9.

38 White CB. Smoothing out transitions: how pedagogy influences medical students' achievement of self-regulated learning goals. *Adv Health Sci Ed*. 2007; **12**: 279–97.

CHAPTER 3

Learning to be professional: recent developments in undergraduate medical education

Amanda Howe

Professionalism can be defined as 'a set of values, behaviours, and relationships that underpins the trust the public has in doctors'.[1] This means that learning needs to affect the way that student doctors choose to behave towards patients, colleagues and themselves. Any medical programme now needs to set clear professional outcomes and develop students' motivation and ability to attain these. The General Medical Council (GMC) is the regulator for medical qualifications and licensing in the United Kingdom, and their documentation makes it clear that medical schools should teach, assess and judge student professionalism.[2,3] This is a relatively recent development, with the bulk of literature being less than two decades old.[4,5] Historically, medicine was taught by example in an apprenticeship setting, with the emphasis on the acquisition and application of scientific knowledge and clinical expertise in a biomedical model.[6] Traditional curricula and methods often did not support professionalism, leaving the risk that students might pass on academic grounds but perform poorly in professional domains. While scandals such as the murders committed by Harold Shipman[7] are relatively few, poor communication, laziness, unsafe practices and addictions are all relatively common reasons for doctors to be reported to the GMC.

Learning to be professional is not just a matter of applying appropriate knowledge and skills, but also an integration of the 'what' and 'how' with the 'who' – so that students not only know what is and is not a professional way to behave, but also how to manage their own relationships, emotions and values to achieve the best ends for patients. The challenges of learning to be professional are therefore considerable, as are those involved in assessing student progress: the contextual relevance of one's actions clearly makes the justification for finding someone's behaviour unprofessional more complex than an assessment of their factual accuracy and technical skills.[8] This may especially be true in the stage before direct judgements about behaviour with patients can be assessed – in most medical schools, students will be judged on 'proxy' behaviours such as prompt compliance with academic deadlines and avoidance of plagiarism. The extent to which such behaviours really reflect professional values and attitudes can also be questioned, especially when students are novices and may be unfamiliar with some of the issues of concern.[9] Nevertheless, there is now a strong degree of consensus that learning about, becoming responsible for, and being assessed on, one's professional values and behaviours should start early in medical training.[10] This chapter therefore assumes that our task in undergraduate medical education is to enable each student to graduate with an effective professional persona,[1] and gives an overview of the types of learning methods and assessment that can effectively underpin this development.

Let us look at a brief narrative of a typical medical student's pathway in learning to be professional – they may gain their image of medical practice from their own experiences of healthcare, their family members' experiences as patients or practitioners, media images, or from the aspirations of their teachers. When researching possible university choices, they will get information from documentation (electronic and hard copy), and from work experiences and peer discussion. So the first image of medical professionalism that universities can influence is likely to be through their admissions documentation and selection process. Statements about their expectations of students (*see* Box 3.1), handling declarations of criminal disclosure, content of interviews and staff attitudes in customer contact all set a 'tone' where medical schools can start to make explicit their cultural assumptions of their future novice professionals.

BOX 3.1 Example of an admissions brochure statement*

'The . . . MB/BS is a professional qualification, and all our students need to develop themselves as professionals during the course. In general, our students rise to this challenge: they are hardworking, reliable, patient-centred, appreciative and supportive of others, try to improve things that could be better, and learn fast from any problems. We reward good progress in professionalism on an annual basis by a recognised 'pass' in this area, which can be declared in your CV, and exceptional achievement may also be recognised over time. However we have seen some problems arise.

So to those applying we want you to know that all students of the UEA MB/BS are expected to:

1 Comply with the spirit and principles set out by the accrediting body, the General Medical Council (*see* www.gmc.org.uk)
2 Ensure patient safety and well-being in every way you can
3 Be honest and truthful in all areas of your interaction with staff, other students and patients (in admissions, your UCAS statements must be truthful)
4 Be responsible about all formal requirements (for incoming students, this includes declaration of all problems, e.g. disabilities, criminal records)
5 Be respectful of the needs and efforts of others
6 Seek help when needed
7 Protect the reputation of the medical school.

Our students start working with their peers and patients very early on. We judge your professionalism through an extensive set of behaviours across your work in the University and in clinical settings. This means that we are serious about professionalism! We model all our procedures on those expected of you after qualifying. By the end of your course with us you will already be equipped to behave appropriately with patients and colleagues, and to be really respected for your self-conduct. Start here.'

* www.uea.ac.uk/med/course/mbbs/fitness (accessed 1.6.2010)

On admission, the first weeks of the course will be taken up with institutional process, and adjusting to a new living and learning environment. Specific lectures, signed learning contracts and early patient contact[11] can all be used to make the expectations and context of the course around professionalism clear to the students, as well as further references to professionalism and fitness to practise in core handbooks and documentary guidance. However, the bulk of student activity in the early years of a course will be around the learning of core clinical method and supporting scientific knowledge – so learning to be professional risks being marginalised unless it is embedded into the core curriculum. Common ways of doing this include:

➤ inclusion of professional learning outcomes in problem-based learning and simulated patient cases – for example, a patient with dyspepsia can be the focus of learning about respect for their autonomy (lifestyle or medication choices), the inverse care law (why patients who push for early referral may not be those who need it most) and teamwork (the role of practice nurses in triage), as well as cellular pathology and diagnostics

➤ consistent expectations of students' own professionalism – attendance, punctuality, respect for others, meeting deadlines, high standard of work

➤ emphasis on giving and getting feedback, learning from others, and working in teams; and

➤ specific use of consultation skills, patient contact, ethics and humanities, learning to develop students' ability to develop their skills to reflect and critique situations where there is uncertainty about the best course of action and outcome, or where there is likely to be significant societal prejudice.[12]

As students advance in the course, their skills in professional competence should reach a level where their ability to deliberate and apply principles to new situations in a more subtle and effective manner becomes embedded into their daily practice.[13] Additional ways of learning these professional skills are reflection on and analysis of significant events;[14] analysis of variations in performance (audit or quality improvement initiatives); and self-analysis with review of feedback. These are examples of more sophisticated educational processes, whereby individual students are encouraged to scrutinise their assumptions about patients' needs, and make this part of their conscious professional repertoire.[15] The aim of this aspect of the course is to enable them increasingly to be aware of and command their own reactions, in order to use their own personality effectively in clinical relationships and encounters. Many clinical tutors lack experience and understanding of the importance of this kind of learning opportunity, but there is clear evidence that setting aside the time and personal attention to thinking through complex issues enable students to both unburden feelings and gain 'metacognitive' abilities to assist in rigorous analysis.

So, the motivated medical school can ensure that students are moved through a combination of suitable educational activities that are relevant to facilitation of learning professional expectations and attitudes.[16] But to ensure that these are effective there must also be both formative and summative assessment of their learning. Our student is therefore likely to be asked to reflect on their own professionalism by:

➤ considering the feedback they get from peers and tutors – both routine feedback or that offered as a consequence of perceived problems
➤ writing up complex cases, significant events and important experiences, especially those with some emotional or ethical complexity such as care of the dying, or the doctor as patient
➤ completing assignment tasks in social sciences and humanities, which may have specific focus on issues around the exercise of power, societal diversity, or the role of doctors in society
➤ taking responsibility for any behavioural problems such as non-attendance, late submission of work, impacts of personal stressors, and problems with others; and
➤ acceptance of the school's fitness to practise progression requirements.

Whether they are able to utilise these learning opportunities effectively depends in part on the student's own prior experiences and personality,[17] and in part on the organisational and interpersonal influences they perceive during these important formative years. Crucial to this are the role models they encounter.[18] So alongside the strengthening of student professionalism, all schools need to run a really strong organisational leadership programme to bring out the best in its clinical tutors.[19] Use of community settings, where patients are in their own surroundings and clinical methods are more patient-centred, are also known to motivate students' developing professionalism, as are student-centred relationships with tutors and teams.[20]

Even then, the outcomes of learning professionalism are unpredictable because of the potential variation of input by the student, course, peers, patients and staff. Systematic organisational approaches which model professionalism, value students, reward good behaviour and remediate problems early are likely to be important in avoiding the historical problems of increasing cynicism and negativity in student doctors.[21] Consistency of learning opportunities and fairness in criticism is important to enhancing rather than demotivating students: schools need to accept student scrutiny and feedback with the same professionalism that they expect of students. Similarly, a genuine will from faculty to develop students through every possible learning opportunity is crucial to the successful outcome of a more explicit approach to the learning of professionalism. This needs to include personal human engagement with the student for whom past or present life events threaten to derail their passage through the course.

This takes us to the greatest challenges to learning to be professional, which even some of the most innovative medical programmes have not yet fully addressed. Students in medicine will meet the dying, the abused, the homeless, the addicted and the inadequate, as well as the sick and the healthy. They may themselves experience concurrent difficulties in relationships or health; may have had traumatic experiences that are restimulated by these contacts; or may have other less overt personal issues that the challenges of medicine may reveal. Working with someone to overcome significant health or psychological barriers to their professional development is a skilled job best passed on to trained professionals, but schools need senior staff who can utilise modest therapeutic skills to support students in difficulties until these resolve, they take up referral, or formal fitness to practise procedures have to be instigated. Although this may seem peripheral to teaching and learning, there is a need for a managed cascade of diagnosis and management for students in difficulties that sustains (and eventually enhances) their educational performance wherever possible. Peers, tutors and student support services will be crucial to avoiding academic failure while a student works through illness and personal difficulty, or learns the difficult lessons about how goodwill alone is not enough to qualify a professional. Staff and students will watch and learn from humane and professional role models as they see senior staff negotiate the difficult boundaries of confidentiality, evidence gathering, investigation and remediation. They will also be the witnesses when the school makes a judgement that a student's professionalism is inadequate for graduation, and will scrutinise those judgements. Such judgements test what it means to be professional and brings into sharp focus our integrity, compassion, principles and evidence.

Having given an overview of the learning approaches to professional development that may occur in the modern curriculum, the second half of this chapter will focus on some specific examples of recent developments. These are the use of portfolios to assist reflective learning from experience and monitoring of lapses in professionalism. These have been selected because they align with important pedagogical developments requested from literature reviews earlier this decade,[22] but they appear less common in the recent literature than some of the approaches already mentioned in this chapter.

Portfolio-based learning is 'a widely used method of bringing together a disparate set of educational activities that require self-directedness and reflexivity',[23] and can be used to explore and moderate student responses to professional challenges that might otherwise remain hidden and could block development.[24] Portfolios also require the student to make recurrent input, and to be able to summarise and organise material for selective presentation. Many medical schools now use some kind of portfolio of learning activities to both encourage reflection on specific experiences and also to monitor and mentor students. Some possibilities are summarised in Table 3.1, and schools will have to make choices about exactly how to utilise these. What is clear from emerging work is that reflective writing can reveal weaknesses in student engagement with experience, and can identify the few students who find reflective self-examination difficult, or who resist such professional activities.[25]

One component of a portfolio can relate to longitudinal collation of feedback received from others, and this can complement formal academic monitoring by allowing tutors to inspect student progression in order to strengthen specific learning needs.[26] At UEA we have instituted a student-held record which students must discuss on an annual basis with their personal advisers, and which combines an academic record with career and personal issues that the student wishes to review. Problematic feedback passed to the tutor for remediation can be raised by either party at the same review. This can then also lead into reflective essay writing later in the year, from which learning goals lead back into the annual review.

Few schools have as yet reported the outcomes of their professionalism

TABLE 3.1 Possible aspects of portfolios for professional development

What does it involve?	Needs assessment	Methods	Products	Assessment
Decision on purpose of portfolio	Learning profile	Reflective diary	Articles read and critiqued	Match to defined objectives
Essential elements to include	Necessities	Reading notes from tutorials	Audits completed	Evidence of outcomes
Acceptable format	Opportunities	Audit	Protocols prepared	Summary of activities
Stages and timescale of preparation/ submission	Strengths and weaknesses	Career review	Written case study	Standard of product
Monitoring of progress	Workload diary	Peer discussion	Events attended	Certificates of attendance
Mentoring or support	Critical incidents	Shadowing	Presentations	Verification of claims from third parties
Mode of accreditation	Case studies → learning plan		Content of tutorials	Specific examination of components, e.g. log book
			Feedback summary	
			Results summary	

teaching in terms of quantitative descriptors. In Table 3.2, there is a summary of the behaviours monitored within the teaching and learning context, and how problems may be reported. In a 6-year period it was found that only 15% of students had any problems at all in a professionalism domain: most of these presented either via absence from teaching or via tutors who were concerned about weak work, plagiarism, or poor interpersonal relationships. This again points up the intimate link between the learning encounter and the potency of this setting to detect, diagnose and remediate professionalism issues. So even if the declarative purpose of a learning event is around core science, it is important that a tutor (especially one who sees a student recurrently over a period of time) is given encouragement, responsibility and the tools to assess a student from a professional perspective.

Students in the modern health service need to learn to work with others, both patients and staff, from other disciplines. This has been particularly highlighted around safe practice issues,[27] but there can be resistance between different professional student groups as cultures clash and new identities are

TABLE 3.2 Examples of behaviours monitored for professionalism purposes

Behaviour	Reporting route
• Honesty – including avoidance of plagiarism, or falsification (e.g. signatures)	• Via assessors or tutors to Course Director
	• Tutor reports
• Respect – including cultural difference	• Peer reports
• Is fair, does not show prejudice	
• Taking responsibility	
• Teamwork	
• Attendance and timeliness	• Attendance registers
• Meeting institutional requirements	• Reports from staff detecting problem
• Other behaviours giving staff or peers cause for significant concerns	• Staff or student concern form (verbal reports confirmed in writing)

formed.[28] The consistent building in to medical courses of learning events where different students meet is still rare, but is strongly advocated both by Government mindful of future workforce needs and by schools who see this as a professional priority. At UEA we have a course running over the first three years which allows students from medicine, nursing, pharmacy and allied health to work through shared case studies, meet different staff members, and compare their different roles in clinical care. This complements the teaching they receive in the NHS from many staff members of different professional backgrounds. Again, this is linked with their portfolio by making 'teamwork' the specific theme of the summative reflective essay in year 2.

There are many other examples where professionalism is tested – in community placements and electives with agencies which work in partnership with medicine; in routine clinical contacts where patient encounters bring crucial challenges to students around their ability to build trust and communicate effectively; in unforeseen circumstances where students may have to assist in emergencies and show their own preparedness and nerve. The readers will be able to populate this chapter with their own experiences. What matters most is not whether students can give a rehearsed answer to how and when they learned to be professional – but more their overall willingness to engage with this task within and outwith the course. Ultimately, the judgement of our teaching and learning is the kind of doctors they become (or not).

REFERENCES

1 Royal College of Physicians. *Doctors in Society: medical professionalism in a changing world.* Report of a Working Party of the Royal College of Physicians of London. London: RCP; 2005.

2 General Medical Council. *Tomorrow's Doctors,* 2nd edn. London: GMC; 2009.

3 General Medical Council. *Medical Students: professional values and fitness to practise.* London: GMC; 2009.

4 Howe A. Professional development in undergraduate medical curricula: the key to the door of a new culture. *Med Educ.* 2002; **36**: 353–9.

5 Howe A. Twelve tips for developing professional attitudes in training. *Med Teach.* 2003; **25**(5): 485–7.

6 Weatherall D. *Science and the Quiet Art: medical research and patient care.* Oxford: Oxford Medical Publications; 1997.

7 www.the-shipman-inquiry.org.uk/ (accessed 12.12.2009)

8 Ginsburg S, Regehr G, Hatala R *et al.* Context, conflict, and resolution: a new conceptual framework for evaluating professionalism. *Acad Med.* 2000; **75**(10 suppl): S6–S11.

9 Rees CE, Knight LV. The trouble with assessing students' professionalism: theoretical insights from sociocognitive psychology. *Acad Med.* 2007; **82**(1): 46–50.

10 Levenson R, Dewar S, Shepherd S. *Understanding Doctors: harnessing professionalism.* King's Fund: London; 2008.

11 Hopayian K, Howe A, Dagley V. A survey of UK medical schools' arrangements for early patient contact. *Med Teach.* 2008; **29**: 806–13.

12 Batson CD, Polycarpou MP, Harmon-Jones E *et al.* Empathy and attitudes: can feeling for a member of a stigmatized group improve feelings towards the group? *J Personality & Soc Psychol.* 1997; **7**(1): 105–18.

13 Eraut M. *Developing Professional Knowledge and Competence.* London: Falmer Press; 1994.

14 Henderson E, Hogan H, Grant A *et al.* Undergraduate learning. Conflict and coping strategies: a qualitative study of student attitudes to significant event analysis. *Med Educ.* 2003; **37**(5): 433–48.

15 Eraut M. Non-formal learning and tacit knowledge in professional work. *Br J Educ Psychol.* 2000; **70**: 113–36.

16 Maudsley G, Strivens J. Promoting professional knowledge, experiential learning and critical thinking for medical students. *Med Educ.* 2000; **34**: 535–44.

17 Enns MW, Cox BJ, Jitsander J *et al.* Adaptive and maladaptive perfectionism in medical students: a longitudinal investigation. *Med Educ.* 2001; **35**: 1034–42.

18 Paice E, Heard S, Moss F. How important are role models in making good doctors? *BMJ.* 2002; **325**: 707–10.

19 Bleakley A. Pre-registration house officers and ward-based learning. *Med Educ.* 2002; **36**: 9–15.

20 Howe A. Patient-centred medicine through student-centred teaching: a student perspective on the key impacts of community-based learning in undergraduate medical education. *Med Educ.* 2001; **35**: 666–72.

21 Rezler A. Attitude changes during medical school: a review of the literature. *J Med Educ.* 1974; **49**: 1023–30.

22 Arnold L. Assessing professional behavior: yesterday, today, and tomorrow. *Acad Med.* 2002; **77**: 502–15.

23 Snadden D, Thomas M. The use of portfolios in medical education. *Med Teach.* 1998; **20**: 192–9.

24 Phillips C. Student portfolios and the hidden curriculum on gender: mapping exclusion. *Med Educ.* 2009; **43**: 821–925.

25 Howe A, Barrett A, Leinster S. How medical students demonstrate their professionalism when reflecting on experience. *Med Educ.* 2009; **43**: 942–51.

26 Cleary L. 'Forward feeding' about students' progress: the case for longitudinal, progressive, and shared assessment of medical students. *Acad Med.* 2008; **83**(9): 800.

27 Howe A. Can the patient be on our team? An operational approach to patient involvement in interprofessional approaches to safe care. *J Interprof Care.* 2006; **20**(5): 527–34.

28 Roberts C, Howe A, Winterburn S *et al.* 'Not so easy as it sounds' – study of a shared learning project between medical and nursing undergraduate students. *Med Teach.* 2000; **22**(4): 386–91.

CHAPTER 4

A personal perspective on the curriculum shift from traditional to PBL, etc.

Sam J Leinster

Change, it is said, is the only constant in medical education. The drivers for change are diverse. At one level is the need to respond to the development of scientific knowledge and the consequent changes to clinical practice. At another level, there are changes in societal attitude reflected in ethical debate, legal enactment and funding decisions. More recently a major driver has been the growing engagement of medical educators with educational theory and consequent attempts to apply these to the delivery of medical education. Most of the time the change is evolutionary and incremental but from time-to-time more rapid and widespread change takes place. Such a period of rapid change occurred in the UK in the early 1990s in response to the General Medical Council's (GMC) publication of their recommendations for undergraduate medical education, *Tomorrow's Doctors* (1993),[1] and the aftershocks are still being felt.

When *Tomorrow's Doctors* was published, the University of Liverpool Medical School was already in the process of major curriculum review. As it happened, the direction of change under debate concurred with the GMC recommendations. The appearance of *Tomorrow's Doctors* sanctioned the need for change and affirmed the proposals under discussion. The process of change took longer than expected and for practical administrative reasons the new curriculum was not implemented until September 1996.

In 1999, the Medical Workforce Standing Advisory Committee recommended that the number of doctors trained in England and Wales should be increased by 1000. The following year this was increased by a further 1000, making an overall increase of 20%. A Joint Implementation Group (JIG) was set up between the Department of Health and the Higher Education Funding Council for England (HEFCE) to oversee the process of establishing medical school places to cater for the increase. They invited bids for extra student numbers from established schools but also agreed to the creation of new medical schools for the first time in over 30 years.[2] Four medical schools were created *de novo* and three further schools were created in partnership with existing schools (*see* Table 4.1).

TABLE 4.1 Medical Schools founded since 1999

Medical School	Host University	Partner University
Durham	University of Durham	University of Newcastle
Keele	University of Keele	University of Manchester
Warwick	University of Warwick	University of Leicester
Peninsula	University of Exeter and University of Plymouth	
East Anglia	University of East Anglia	
Brighton–Sussex	University of Brighton and University of Sussex	
Hull–York	University of Hull and University of York	

PERSONAL EXPERIENCE

I had the unusual experience of being involved in the development and implementation of the reformed curriculum in Liverpool and subsequently leading the development and implementation of the new curriculum at the University of East Anglia (UEA). The setting of the two schools is different. The University of Liverpool is one of the Victorian 'red-brick'

Universities and was founded in 1881. The medical school pre-dates the University and was founded in 1834, becoming the Faculty of Medicine of the then University College, Liverpool in 1884. Liverpool is the fourth largest city in the UK and is surrounded by the Liverpool Urban Area giving a conurbation with a population of over 800 000. Along with the Metropolitan Borough of Wirral, on the opposite bank of the River Mersey, it forms the metropolitan county of Merseyside with a population of over 1.3 million.[3] The University of East Anglia was founded in 1964 as part of the expansion of higher education in the UK that followed the Robbins Report.[4] It is situated on the outskirts of Norwich which is an ancient cathedral city with a population of 120 000 set in one of the most rural and sparsely populated parts of England. There are marked differences in health profiles between the two regions. The life expectancy in Liverpool is 73 years for males and 78 years for females; in Norfolk it is 78 years and 82 years respectively.[5]

The overall educational and philosophical outlook of the teams involved in these curricula was similar. Both groups fully espoused the recommendations of the GMC with regard to identification of a core curriculum, integration of theory and practice and the introduction of early clinical contact. In each case the core curriculum was defined by a series of index cases (200 in the case of Liverpool; 150 in the case of UEA). Both groups chose to use problem-based learning (PBL) as the principal mode of delivering learning supported by lectures and seminars.

In Liverpool, the new curriculum had to be delivered to the new intake of students while the students in the remaining 4 years of the course continued on the old curriculum. Resource constraints, particularly in clinical placements, meant that early clinical contact had to be restricted. During the first year the 'clinical' component was based in the Clinical Skills Laboratory and comprised history taking, clinical examination and some practical skills. This was supplemented by communication skills sessions using small group tutorials and role play. The first contact with real patients occurred in the second year and took place in primary care practices and hospitals throughout the city. The structure of the curriculum from Year 3 onwards was partly dictated by which clinical placements were free to take the students. This problem did not arise at UEA. A small number of students from the medical schools in London and Cambridge undertook placements in the Norfolk and Norwich and James Paget Hospitals but effectively placements could be planned at any stage of the curriculum without the constraints of adjusting for other groups of students.

THE LIVERPOOL EXPERIENCE

At Liverpool there was an established infrastructure for undergraduate medical education. Each discipline taught in the curriculum was represented by a department headed by a senior academic, usually a Professor, and staffed by a substantial complement of lecturers and senior lecturers. For many years the curriculum content in each subject was decided primarily by the department and delivered by that department. The curriculum was divided into distinct pre-clinical and clinical phases with little patient contact during the pre-clinical phase. Even within the phases there was little integration between departments. Curriculum reform was attempted on a number of occasions without any fundamental change resulting.

In 1989, it was decided that another attempt should be made to introduce reform. Debate took place around the reason for the limited success of previous attempts. It was clear that change could only occur if departmental heads agreed that it was needed. However, the existing faculty structures were predicated on the current curriculum. Extensive change could lead to changes in the staffing needs of faculty with a major impact on the staffing of each department. There was a real risk of such change impacting on a department's research capability. There was therefore a risk that department heads would be reluctant to contemplate radical change. It was thought that more junior members of staff with an active interest in medical education would be more likely to consider radical change. Previous experience suggested that it would be difficult to persuade the faculty to accept their recommendations.

It was apparent that there were four steps to achieving change. The first step was to persuade faculty of the need for change. The second was to identify the changes that needed to take place. The third was to plan the introduction of change, and the fourth was to implement the change. The solution was to establish two committees. The *Curriculum Strategy Group* (CSG) comprised the heads of department of Anatomy, Medicine and Primary Care, plus a Senior Lecturer in Surgery (the current author) who had a special interest in medical education. The Senior Lecturer in Surgery chaired the *Curriculum Design Group* (CDG) that was drawn from Lecturers and Senior Lecturers in the major departments.

The role of the CSG was to agree the need for change and identify the principles on which curriculum change should be based. The CDG was then tasked with interpreting the principles and specifying the exact nature of the changes. The proposed changes were based on educational theory supported by international examples of good practice. For efficiency, the main work of the CDG was carried out by an inner core of four people. These were the Senior Lecturer in Surgery, a Senior Lecturer in Medicine, a Lecturer in Anatomy and a medical educationalist with a background in general practice. While the first three were seconded from their departments, the fourth was employed specifically to facilitate the process. The 'gang of four' as it became known met on a weekly basis to discuss plans and progress, and to agree tasks.

The CSG agreed that the course would be built around four main themes:

➤ Structure and function
➤ Individuals, groups and society
➤ Population perspective
➤ Professional values and personal development.

From the beginning it was agreed that the course should be integrated vertically (pre-clinical with clinical) and horizontally (between disciplines). It was also accepted that there had to be a reduction in the factual content with an increased emphasis on the development of intellectual and cognitive skills. The CDG concluded that the first could best be achieved by adopting problem-based learning (PBL)[6] as the main educational tool. There was a lot of debate about how the second could be achieved while ensuring that students learnt the essentials of medicine. An important concept that informed the debate was the idea that clinical reasoning is based on the use of *cognitive schemata* or *scripts*.[7] This led to the proposal that the curriculum should be based around a number of *index cases*, a concept that was developed simultaneously but independently in Calgary[8] and Manchester.[9]

A separate group was set up with the task of deciding on the index cases. The group was co-chaired by the Professor of Immunology and a Senior Lecturer in General Practice. Each department or discipline had a representative. Each member of the group was invited to suggest their own *core cases* and each list was then debated by the whole group until an agreed list was produced. This list was then sent to a wide range of clinicians in the region with a request for comment and editing. The returned comments were collated and the list was modified by the group and again sent out for comment. Following this iteration the final list was agreed and formed the basis for defining the core curriculum. Nothing could appear in the curriculum unless it related to one of the core cases.

Meanwhile, the CDG was discussing the structure of the curriculum. A fifth member had joined the group who proved to be invaluable at this stage of the planning. In response to the GMC's recommendations for reform in *Tomorrow's Doctors*, the Chief Medical Officer for England had provided funding to pay for *curriculum facilitators* in each medical school. Liverpool employed a non-medical educationalist with extensive experience in secondary school education. He brought an understanding of the need for a transparent structure for the curriculum. In response, the CDG decided on a curriculum that would have three phases. In the first phase (occupying the first year) the students would be given an introduction to medical science and practice. The second phase occupied Years 2–4 and was divided into Phase 2a: Normal Structure and Function, and Phase 2b: Pathophysiology. The final year was Phase 3 and provided intensive clinical experience.

The *core cases* were arranged according to where they would most likely present chronologically in the life cycle. Typical cases were selected for each stage of the life cycle and these were used to develop scenarios for the problem-based tutorials for each phase. Phase 1 then started at conception and moved through the clinical cases until old age and death. Phase 2a started again at conception but considered the normal structure and function relating to the cases in greater depth. Phase 2b started again at conception but considered the abnormalities that could arise at each stage. Each phase was then split into a number of modules based on single PBL scenarios, each of which occupied two weeks of curricular time. Once the theoretical backbone had been developed the timetable for the concurrent clinical experience was planned.

While the two curriculum groups worked well and effectively together, we recognised that acceptance of such radical change would depend on the whole faculty feeling ownership of the project. There was a manifest tension between the need to involve as many people as possible to achieve ownership and the utility of maintaining a small group to achieve efficiency.

The solution was devolution of responsibility for the detailed development of the curricular content. Phase Groups were appointed to manage each phase. They managed a series of modular groups, each of which was responsible for developing the detailed content of a case-based scenario. Other members of faculty were given specific responsibility for ensuring that the themes were adequately represented throughout the curriculum. Given that four to five individuals were engaged with each module it is obvious that a considerable number of faculty were actively engaged in curriculum development. Maintaining a consistent approach in line with the agreed principles required major efforts in communication between the different levels.

At another level departments were engaged by a series of visits by members of the CDG explaining the developments as they took place and entering into dialogue with the departmental staff. Formal communication with faculty took place through regular reports to the Board of Faculty who had to approve each stage of the planning. The management of the presentations to the Board was an important part of the change process. As each decision was agreed by the CSG and the CDG it was presented to the Board for approval. The next stage could then be presented as the logical outcome of the steps that had already been approved. Members of the Board had the opportunity to adjust to and accept the changes incrementally rather than being faced with agreeing to a sudden paradigm shift.

THE UEA EXPERIENCE

The process at UEA was different in many ways. When the medical school was first proposed in 1999 there was no one with any experience of developing or managing an undergraduate medical curriculum, although the University had an established School of Occupational and Physiotherapy and a School of Nursing and Midwifery. A small project group was formed which comprised the Pro-Vice Chancellor for the Health Schools (a Clinical Psychologist by profession) and a group of NHS consultants and general practitioners. They were supported by a senior administrator, seconded by the University, to help prepare the bid documentation. The established health schools had a shared philosophy that included the integration of theory and practice; problem-orientated learning; an emphasis on interprofessional learning; and clinical placements in a variety of settings including primary care. The project group decided that the medical curriculum would follow the same principles.

They sought advice from the University of Manchester and, most significantly, from the University of Calgary. They decided that they would adopt the *index case* approach and structure the course in system-based modules. Professor Henry Mandin from Calgary agreed to provide significant input to the development of the curriculum and spent 3 months in Norwich working with the project group to produce an outline curriculum for presentation to the *Joint Implementation Group* of the Department of Health and the Department of Education. The list of clinical presentations from Calgary was revised by the local clinicians to ensure that it was consistent with the local disease profile.

By the time that the bid was submitted, the curriculum had a clear structure that had similarities to the Calgary curriculum but had significant differences. The most obvious difference was the loss of the pre-clinical/clinical divide which had been an important feature of medical education since the adoption of the Flexner Report in 1910.[10] In the UEA curriculum, clinical placements begin in the first year and the basic sciences continue to be taught until the end of the final year. Each body system is represented by a single module. Campus-based teaching occupies two-thirds of each module with placement in secondary care making up the other third. Throughout the course the students spend one day a week in primary care during the campus-based component of the curriculum. The proposed method of learning was based on Calgary's *Clinical Presentations* curriculum. An important step was the development of a *Curriculum Framework* which established the topics and disciplines that had to be covered in considering each case. The framework was classified into broad subject categories that were then sub-divided into disciplines or themes (*see* Table 4.2). It was expected that learning outcomes would be generated for each case using the framework to verify that all the important topics had been covered. One module was worked out in detail as part of the bid process.

Once the Joint Implementation Group gave approval for the formation of a new medical school, the University sought to appoint a Dean with an interest in medical education and experience of curriculum development. The author was successful in obtaining the post and joined the project group in January 2001.

TABLE 4.2 Curriculum framework

Clinical	Individual patient Family/community Population
Life sciences	Anatomy/histology/diagnostic imaging Biochemistry Genetics Immunology Microbiology Pathology Pharmacology Physiology
Socio-economic aspects	Ethics Law Health economics Health service management Psychology Sociology
Skills	Clinical skills Consultation skills Inter-professional skills IT Organisational skills
Settings	Primary care Secondary and tertiary care Public health
Student	Personal and professional development

The next stage of the process was a negotiation between the new Dean and the rest of the project group with regard to the final form of the curriculum. For both theoretical and practical reasons, the Dean wished to introduce PBL in a formula similar to Liverpool's rather than the Calgary Clinical Presentations approach. There was considerable agreement on the structure of the curriculum, particularly the early clinical placements; the emphasis on primary care; and the defining of the core curriculum through index cases. There was total agreement on the philosophy of the course that placed as much emphasis on the psychosocial and population sciences as on the biological sciences. The fact that the Dean had practical experience of delivering a PBL curriculum swayed the decision and the mode of delivery was altered.

In a process similar to that employed in Liverpool, Module Teams were appointed to develop each of the system-based modules. However, unlike Liverpool, there were limited numbers of academic staff. For that reason, interested NHS consultants and general practitioners were recruited to the task. The importance of the role was recognised by them being given specific sessions in their job plans for the undertaking. Academic staff were gradually recruited and each module was given an academic lead as they became available. The process was co-ordinated by the project group that gradually evolved into the Curriculum Design and Delivery Group (CDD) as individuals with new expertise joined the school.

An early task for the Module Teams was confirming that the index cases assigned to their module were appropriate. The list from the bid was compared with the lists from Liverpool and Manchester. A further check was made against the cases that form the basis of the GMC's Professional and Linguistics Board test, which in turn were derived from hospital and general practitioner statistics. The final list contained 150 cases. The differences in the number of cases between the various lists are due to variations in the extent to which symptoms are combined or split. The actual range of conditions is remarkably similar.

The team then examined the cases and decided on the learning outcomes that applied. The learning outcomes were then used to develop the scenarios for the PBL cases and to decide on the lectures and seminars that would be delivered.

One of the challenges was ensuring that all of the core material was covered and that it developed in an ordered and logical way across the 5 years. Academic staff were appointed according to a pre-agreed schedule which depended on the gradually increasing income of the school from student numbers. As discipline specialists joined the team they were given responsibility of taking an overview of their subjects within the curriculum. Their proposals were brought back to the CDD to verify that the scope and level of the proposed learning outcomes had the agreement of the rest of the team.

As the school was new, the GMC appointed an inspection team to oversee its development. The interaction between the GMC and the school was an important element in the progress of the curriculum. The constant discussion with a group of critical friends helped to identify the strengths and weaknesses of the proposals. For example, there were disagreements around the original assessment policy of the school that did not include a final examination. Readiness for graduation was to be decided by a review of the student's performance throughout the entire course. The whole policy was revised in the light of the debate; the overall assessment burden was reduced and a new format of finals was devised. The regular inspections of teaching events and examinations helped to reassure the student body that their qualifications were equivalent to those of other schools.

COMPARING THE EXPERIENCES

The engagement of the local clinicians was essential to the success of the venture in both schools. In Liverpool, there was a well-established network of *Clinical Sub-Deans* in each of the hospitals engaged in teaching. This group was made responsible for informing and recruiting the clinicians in their own hospital. They formed local committees within the hospitals who were responsible for developing the teaching programme within that locality in line with the principles and learning outcomes laid down by the CDG. At UEA, there was no established network. Some clinicians had been instrumental in establishing the school but others were anxious about the impact that the existence of the school would have on medical practice in the area. Presentations to large groups of clinicians at specially organised meetings were supplemented with attendance at the regular divisional meetings of specialty groups within the local hospitals. The clinicians in the hospitals who were already engaged as part of the team who bid for the medical school were an important part of the process as they acted as guarantors of the legitimacy of the proposals. This was necessary as the medical school team were unknown within the local health economy. In particular, no one was familiar with their clinical credentials and there was a tendency to regard them as 'medical educators' divorced from the exigencies of real-life practice. This contrasted with Liverpool where the main protagonists were known and respected as practising clinicians.

The potential result of failure to implement the proposed curriculum was different in the two cases. In Liverpool, a functioning curriculum was in place. Failure to implement the new curriculum would have resulted in embarrassment for the group leading the process, but the medical school could have continued to deliver an undergraduate programme using the existing curriculum. Some investment was made in buildings and other fixed resources to meet the needs of the new programme but these facilities could have been used for the existing programme and would not have represented a complete loss. The University would have sustained minor financial loss associated with the costs of the project but the income stream from teaching would have continued unchanged. At UEA, there was no fallback position. Failure to implement the curriculum would have meant the loss of the proposed income stream. Alternative sources of funding would have had to be found for the building and resource developments that had been undertaken in expectation of the new income. It is not clear where this would have come from as it is unlikely that the HEFCE would have permitted an equivalent uplift in other student numbers to compensate, especially when the fee level for medical students is considerably higher than for other groups of students.

On the other hand, the rewards for success were much higher at UEA, which had a longstanding ambition to have a medical school. There was considerable interest and support in the community with coverage of the stages of development of the medical school in the local media. In contrast, the curricular changes in Liverpool were of limited interest outside of the medical school itself.

Despite the differences in circumstances there were common factors that contributed to the success. The most important of these was the building of a coherent, committed team with the necessary skills (or the ability to acquire these skills quickly). Both teams had a clear vision of the type of doctor they wanted to produce and a credible plan for how this could be achieved based on a sound understanding of educational theory. Major efforts were made to communicate these plans and the rationale for them to the wider health community who would be responsible for delivering the programme. Both teams were strongly supported by the senior management of the institutions concerned. As a result, the new curriculum was successfully implemented in both cases.

REFERENCES

1 General Medical Council. *Tomorrow's Doctors.* London: GMC; 1993.
2 Bligh J. More medical students for England. *Med Educ.* 2001; **35**: 712–13.

3 Office of National Statistics. www.statistics.gov.uk/census2001/pyramids/pages/2b.asp (accessed 11.5.2010)

4 Department of Health. *The Report of the Robbins Committee on Higher Education*. London: HMSO; 1963.

5 Office of National Statistics. www.statistics.gov.uk/life-expectancy/lifemap.html (accessed 11.5.2010)

6 Bligh J. Problem-based learning in medicine: an introduction. *Postgrad Med J*. 1995; **71**: 323–6.

7 Charlin B, Tarfid J, Boshuizen HPA. Scripts and medical diagnostic knowledge: theory and application for clinical reasoning teaching and research. *Acad Med*. 2000; **75**: 182–90.

8 Mandin H, Harasym P, Eagle C *et al*. Developing a clinical presentation curriculum at the University of Calgary. *Acad Med*. 2000; **75**: 1043–5.

9 O'Neill P, Metcalfe D, David TJ. The core content of the undergraduate curriculum in Manchester. *Med Educ*. 1999; **33**: 470–1.

10 Flexner A. Medical Education in the United States and Canada: a report to the Carnegie Foundation for the Advancement of Teaching. Reproduced in *Bulletin of the World Health Organization*. 2002; **80**(7): 594–602.

CHAPTER 5

The shifting landscape: how undergraduate students have changed

Sandra Gibson and Laura Bowater

The committee holds that unsuitability for a medical career should be the sole barrier to admission to a medical school.[1]

INTRODUCTION

The medical student body has changed markedly since the end of the Second World War. Reforms to medical education and the selection of students into medical training around the mid-20th century, were largely the result of four major events: the centralisation of student number planning; adopting some of the recommendations of the Goodenough Committee; the establishment of the National Health Service as an employer to new graduates; and the introduction of minimum standards of school leaving qualifications.[1,2,3]

Even with the forward thinking recommendations of the Goodenough Committee, advocating that inability to work as a doctor should be the only barrier to studying medicine,[1] the diversity within the English medical student population remained low between the late 1940s and the 1960s.[4] Rather, there was a redistribution of students, for example males and females, resulting in the student population within schools becoming more uniform between medical schools. This redistribution was encouraged by the introduction of public funding to medical schools conditional on schools meeting required student demographic targets set by the University Grants Committee.[5]

A Royal Commission on Medical Education was established in 1968 to address concerns about a lack of home-trained doctors, and the increasing reliance on those from overseas.[6] The recommendation was that the UK should increase its training capacity heralding a period of expansion in the number of places available to study medicine. This increase in capacity facilitated changes in the student population, and coupled with recent initiatives such as the widening participation programmes, facilitated the changes in the overall medical student population that we see today.

In this chapter we present an outline of the main drivers for change in the medical student population over the last 60 years, and how this is reflected in the student population seen on the MB/BS programme at the University of East Anglia (UEA) today.

GENDER

In the 1940s the role of women began to change; societal hierarchies were crumbling, heralding a change to the admittance of females to medical school. Prior to the Goodenough report, the proportion of females attending medical school varied regionally; approximately 20% of medical students in Scotland were female, whereas 75% of London schools admitted men only.[5] The exception to this was the London School of Medicine for Women which had trained women to be doctors since its inception in 1874.[5] The Goodenough report recommended Government financial support to medical schools but this recommendation was reliant on a female admissions quota to all medical schools.[1] It wasn't until after 1947 that all medical schools became co-educational. As a result of this recommendation, women were finally given better access to medical school places. However, strict quotas for female students existed and this was coupled with genuine misgivings about female medical students' ability to succeed as doctors. However, these fears were soon dispelled when females began to outperform male medical students. Conversely, the demand for co-education in medical schools resulted in the admission of male students to the London School of Medicine for Women, which subsequently became the Royal Free Hospital.

In 1963, the Universities and Colleges Admissions Service (UCAS, formerly the Universities Central Council on Admissions (UCCA)) began to collect data on university admissions. It revealed that only 34% of medical school applicants were women and, of those, only 29% were allocated places. These data also showed that admission figures were not uniform across medical schools. Certain medical schools such as the Royal Free had a significant female intake, 61%, while Cambridge had an admissions rate of only 8.5%.[4]

Over the last 15 years there has been a steady increase in the number of females training as doctors. Parity with the male student numbers has been attained and recently exceeded (*see* Figure 5.1).[7,8]

The increase in female admissions that occurred during the 1960s reflects two factors. First, the modernisation of the University admissions procedure into UCCA resulted in an admissions procedure based more on school level

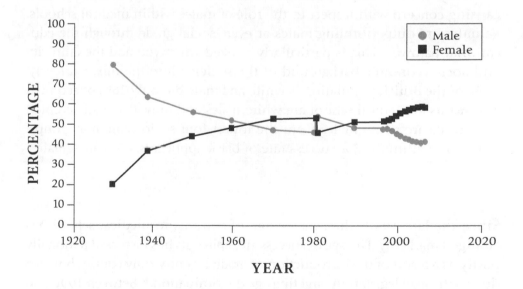

FIGURE 5.1 Percentage of male and female full-time students studying medicine and dentistry between 1930 and 2008. (Data from *Twentieth-Century British Societal Trends*[7] & Higher Education Statistics Agency.[8])

qualifications, rather than individual school set processes.[5] Second, there was an increase in the number of applicants which outstripped the increasing number of available medical school places.[5,6] Increasing medical school places were a result of the Royal Commission on Medical Education,[6] which also highlighted the need for fairer selection procedures. Although the female admission rate increased throughout this period, it has been suggested that this increase was because more female students obtained the school grades required for entry to medical school rather than an active attempt to rectify the gender balance. This view is supported by data showing that the number of female medical students dramatically increased before the introduction of the Gender Equalities Act in 1975.[8] In recent years the number of women applicants and admissions has stabilised at around 60%.[3] Clearly, medicine has become a much more attractive career option for women over the last four decades. The reasons for this are multifactoral but may include a change in the subject choices of females while still at school, increasing grades achieved by females over the same time period, and perhaps the perception that the medical school curriculum has become more female orientated.[3,9]

Many of the changes that have benefited female applicants are now causing concern with respect to the role of males within medical schools. Females are outperforming males at every social grade through the educational pathway. This is particularly marked when you add the ethnicity and socio-economic background of the students into the mix. Currently, 44% of the British population is white and male but only 28% of accepted applicants to medical school are white males and only 4% of all accepted applicants are white males from the lowest four socio-economic groups. Similarly, within the 3% success rate of black applicants, 65% are female.[4]

AGE

Since the late 1940s the average age of entrants to medical school has changed markedly. The age of successful applicants has increased nationally partly as a result of the introduction of graduate entry-only courses but also due to the new legislation targeting age discrimination.[10] Between 1996 and 2009, the number of applying students older than 21 increased dramatically, with the number over 40-years-old increasing five-fold,[4] although in relative terms the number in the older age group is still low. This trend was especially noticeable in the 2003 intake to British medical schools that corresponded to the opening of new medical schools that actively encouraged applications from older students. Presently, there are 16 graduate entry courses, an increase from an initial three in 1999, with additional undergraduate courses also admitting graduates. In addition, there is now a provision of Access to Medicine courses designed for non-traditional, mature students who want to change career in order to study medicine. These courses provide an intensive introduction to the sciences and clearly have a part to play in recruiting older students into medical school.

Although an increase in age of students will enhance diversity and they will bring a wealth of experience to their learning, this may be coupled with an increase of demand on students' time as they balance their work–life relationship.

The UEA Medical School was one of the new medical schools that opened in 2002. The initial two intakes of students had a higher than average proportion of mature students, mainly graduates and those making the transition from other health professions. Since then our student population has stabilised; the average age of our students is currently approximately 21-years-old. This, in part, reflects our diverse student population with approximately 50% of our recent cohorts being school leavers and the rest either graduates or entering through a widening participation route.

ETHNICITY AND NATIONALITY

After the Second World War the vast majority of students were white, male school leavers – the medical workforce today, however, is clearly a multi-ethnic environment. A lot of this multi-ethnicity is due to the influx of oversees trained health workers but it also reflects the proportion of medical students that are now entering and graduating from our medical schools.

In the 1940s there was a wave of political refugees who arrived in the UK throughout the Second World War from countries under German occupation. These refugees included medical students and early career stage doctors who completed their training in the UK. Further immigration into the National Health Service continued after the war and this was in part due to the number of medical school places recommended in a report produced by the Committee on Medical Manpower chaired by Sir Henry Willink.[11] The report was based on the premise that too many doctors were being produced to serve a population that no longer needed such a large medical workforce due to the diminishing of the British Empire and the Armed Forces after the end of the war. Consequently, the report recommended a 10% reduction of medical school places. However, it soon became clear that this recommendation had been a severe underestimation of actual need and the hospital sector began to suffer from a lack of junior doctors. This shortfall resulted in the immigration of overseas doctors into the National Health Service. It also led to the 1961 Platt report commissioned by the Ministry of Health that described the shortage of consultants. As a direct result of this report Mr Enoch Powell, Minister of Health, agreed to a 10% increase in the intake of medical students above the levels recommended in the Willink report. It was agreed that this increase in medical student places could be accommodated in existing university medical schools.[12]

In 1998, an article published in the *British Medical Journal*[13] reported on the different factors that affected applicants being offered a place at medical school. Anonymised information used for this was obtained from UCAS. This study clearly indicated that 'non-white applicants were less likely to receive an offer'.[13] The nationality and ethnic status of students applying to medical school has been relatively stable over the last 7 years, with ≈70% of accepted applicants stating their origin as white, ≈28% non-white and ≈1.9% were unknown.[4] However, it must be noted that the mix of students differs between medical schools. For example, the large, mixed ethnic London population is reflected in the ethnic population of the London medical schools. Of the students that received offers from UEA in 2008, ≈72% did not declare an ethnic group, ≈22% were white and ≈8% were non-white.

An important point to note is that non-white applications are not homogenous. There are distinct differences between ethnic groups entering medical school: in the case of black students it is notable that although the proportion of applicants has increased, the acceptance rate has not. There is also a clear gender difference at play in the figures. Of the 3% of accepted black applicants, 65% of these applicants were female. With reports of black male students underperforming in the school system, it may be that aspirations and educational interventions should be targeted earlier in the educational processes.

Currently, a reduction of funding to higher education has led to universities actively seeking to recruit overseas students, with their associated higher fee paying capacity. This is a trend that can also be seen within medical education. Currently, the number of medical school places that are available for applicants from the UK and European Union remains oversubscribed, but there has been an increase in the number of places for international students.

DISABILITY

It was not until a British Medical Association (BMA) working group report published in 1997[14] that student doctors with a disability were recognised as a group in their own right. This working group was interesting in itself as it contained a significant proportion of members with a disability, a rare occurrence at the time in those advocating disability educational policy.[15] This coincided with the implementation of changes recommended in the Disabilities Discrimination Act 1995 (DDA).[16]

By 2005, the attitude towards recruiting students with disabilities was changing, partly as a response to an amendment to the DDA that required equal opportunities for students with disabilities. As a result, the BMA, General Medical Council (GMC), Quality Assurance Agency (QAA) and Higher Education Authority (HEA), expect medical schools to encourage applications from students with disabilities. They have highlighted that improved information and communication for applicants should be given as the first step. The percentage of students with a disability, accepted into UK medical schools, has risen from 2.8% in 2003 to 3.3% in 2007, in line with the general trend of increasing numbers of students with disabilities in higher education.[4]

In the *Equality and Diversity in UK Medical Schools* report by the BMA,[4] it is clear that although the value of disabled doctors has been recognised, and that students with disabilities have been actively encouraged to apply to medical school, there has been little improvement in the discrimination faced by disabled doctors in the workplace.[4,17,18,19] This issue may well feed into the problem of under reporting of disabilities. Clearly, an environment of openness and willingness to implement reasonable adjustments to accommodate medical students and doctors with disabilities, now a GMC requirement,[20] would begin to reduce this discrimination.

Within the UEA Medical School we have a higher proportion of students than the UK average declaring a disability when compared to medical schools in other universities. The majority of which are specific learning difficulties (SpLDs). We hope that this high number of disabled students reflects a willingness of our students to declare their disability, and that we are attaining the open atmosphere needed to allow students to openly declare their disability.

SOCIAL CLASS (WIDENING PARTICIPATION)

In the mid-20th century, the social diversity of medical schools was slim. The majority of students were white, male school leavers with more than 80% of students originating from professional backgrounds. Although the ethnicity and gender of medical students has changed, the social demographic has remained fairly static over the past five decades.[4,21] Currently, 71% of medical students accepted into medical school are from socio-economic group I (higher managerial and professional occupations), II (lower managerial and professional occupations) and III (intermediate occupations).[4] Currently, just 15% of medical students are from the bottom four social classes, with 2% from the lowest social class indicating a routine manual occupational background. Statistics like these have led to questions about the accessibility of certain professions, such as medicine, to the lower societal groups. In 2009, the Government appointed a panel of experts and representatives from the professions including medicine to look at access to the professions from across society. The report concluded that access to the professions is still focused on families with above average incomes and there is a need to encourage and promote fair access to a medical education. In its document, *Equality and Diversity in UK Medical Schools*,[4] the BMA clearly lays out its support to attract medical students from a broader range of societal backgrounds. The arguments for increasing the diversity of students entering the medical professions express a belief that an increasingly diverse medical population reflects, represents and is best able to meet the needs of a diverse society. There is also a view that increasing the diversity of medical students will ensure that the candidates best suited to a career in medicine are able to become doctors. These opinions have been considered and reflected in *Tomorrow's Doctors*,[20] which emphasises the need for equality and diversity among medical student applicants in the UK. It states that all medical schools should have admission policies 'aimed at ensuring that all applicants and students are treated fairly and have equality of opportunity, regardless of their diverse backgrounds and needs'.[20]

The Government has invested significant funds in promoting widening participation in higher education through schemes such as the Aim Higher programme (2005–06). In 2004, the Higher Education Act agreed to a £3000 a year top-up fee for students. However, this was dependent on a concomitant agreement between Higher Education Institutes (HEIs) and the Office for Fair Access for HEIs to use this additional income to provide bursaries for disadvantaged students, as well as financing outreach initiatives designed to promote widening participation. Despite this focus of energy and resources to encourage students from the lower socio-economic classes into higher education, there appears to have been little success or movement in this area.[21] Participation in higher education among the lower social classes remains stubbornly low despite the investment. This is especially true with applicants to medical school. There is still a perception among pupils from lower social economic groups that medical schools are geared towards affluent students. These pupils greatly underestimate their chances of both gaining a place at medical school and staying the course. It has been suggested that if we are to encourage participation among the lower socio-economic classes to enter medicine, then we must progress from a knowledge deficit model that assumes additional academic support will begin to overturn this imbalance and instead we focus on and address 'the complex social and cultural environment within which individual life choices are embedded' – clearly, a much more difficult proposition.[22] There have been changes to admission procedures to try to address the discrepancies of under-representation in successful applicants to medical school from the lower socio-economic classes and the under-represented groups. Different programmes have been established that legally modify their admission process through the creation of foundation year or widening access programmes that allow entry to medical school from students with lower A level grades or without the required science subjects.

Even in the late 1940s it was apparent that a five-year, and sometimes six-year, medical course was expensive and students from middle class families were struggling to attend the medical schools.[23] The student grant system was brought in where financial support was given to students. However, disincentives were also apparent as any scholarship won was taken off the student grant award.

The length of the medical degree programme and the implementation of top-up fees in the UK over recent years has ensured that studying medicine has become one of the most expensive degree programmes in the UK, with the result that improving access to medicine for students from lower societal backgrounds has an additional hurdle of expense and the consequential high levels of student debt. Recent figures from a national student survey indicate that over 28% of the students who responded expect to graduate with over £20 000 of debt, with parental support being second only to taking out a loan in supporting the students through studies.[24] Of the students surveyed from medicine and allied health subjects, only 26% thought the debt unacceptable.[24] With the recent change in Government planning to implement an increase in student fees, it is clear that parental support and ability to secure a loan will become key issues in determining whether a student would consider applying to study medicine, or being able to continue if financial issues occur during the course.

SUMMARY

There are currently 16 graduate entry courses within the UK and entry to other courses is also open to graduates. These students are thought to bring additional qualities to the role of a doctor. As a result there is now an admissions policy that grants medical studentships to students with additional qualities and not just as a reward for good grades. This admissions policy has also widened the access to medicine by giving opportunities to students who would not have got a place at medical school previously. Within the same timeframe, the grades that are required by students to get into medical school, and the way that places are offered based on the predicted grades of students, has also changed. With recent systems allowing high-predicted grades and greater access to impressive extracurricular activities to students from independent schools, these students appear a more attractive proposition at the selection-for-interview stage. The repercussions of this are a potential bias towards students from independent schools being interviewed and consequently offered medical school places, compared with students from the state sector. Interestingly, evidence is available that shows students from a state school achieve a better degree classification compared to students with similar grades from independent schools.

The first intake of medical students at UEA was in 2002, and the medical school sought to address issues of widening participation. Our first cohort had approximately 20% of students brought in to medicine from non-traditional routes, such as access, foundation courses or previous healthcare experience, and a further 50% were graduates. For cohorts starting in 2002 to 2008, approximately 7% of our students will be 40 or over at the time they graduate. Since then we have increased our widening access student population. Currently, we have approximately 30% of students in this category, a change facilitated by the introduction of a foundation year that actively seeks to recruit students from social classes under-represented in medicine. The average age of our students has lowered to a figure comparable to the national average over the last 3 years, reflecting the stabilisation of our admissions process and increased pool of applicants. Our policy of inclusion is also reflected in our attitude to disabled students, which make up 16.1% of our current student body. This has risen from 13.8% in 2007, which is somewhat higher than the 3.3% that were accepted nationally that year to medical schools. 65% of our students are female, which is comparable with the national average. Because of the high proportion of students reporting their ethnicity as unknown or undeclared, it is difficult to make a valid judgement on ethnicity at this time.

On a final note, it is interesting that the recommendations of the Goodenough Committee still seem relevant today. For example, their recommendation that aptitude testing in addition to interview and exam results should be considered as selection criteria[1] is pertinent to the implementation of multiple mini interviews and psychometric components to entrance examinations, which are designed to test non-cognitive aptitude to study medicine. This helps ensure that medical schools select students on more than their academic ability, and with additional traits that those making the selection believe will make them good doctors.

REFERENCES

1 The Training of Doctors: Report by the Goodenough Committee. *BMJ*. 1944; 2: 121–3.

2 Lambert TW, Goldacre MJ, Parkhouse J. Doctors who qualified in the UK between 1974 and 1993: age, gender, nationality, family status and family formation. *Med Ed*. 1998; 32: 533–7.

3 Drinkwater J, Tullt MP, Dornan T. The effects of gender on medical students' aspirations: a qualitative study. *Med Ed*. 2008; 42: 420–6.

4 British Medical Association. *Equality and Diversity in UK Medical Schools*. London: BMA; 2009.

5 Elston MA. Women doctors in a changing profession: Britain. In: E Riska, K Wegar, editors. *Gender, Work and Medicine: women and the medical division of labour*. London: Sage; 1993.

6 Royal Commission on Medical Education. *1965–68 Report. Cmnd 3569*. London: HMSO; 1968.

7 Halsey AH. Further and higher education. In: AH Halsey, J Webb, editors. *Twentieth-Century British Social Trends*. London: MacMillan Press; 2000.

8 Higher Education Statistic Agency: www.hesa.ac.uk/

9 British Medical Association. *The Demography of Medical Schools: a discussion paper*. London: BMA; 2004.

10 Employment Equality (Age) Regulations 2006. SI 2006 No. 1031. www.opsi.gov.uk/si/si2006/20061031.htm

11 *Report of the Committee to Consider the Future Numbers of Medical Practitioners and the Appropriate Intake of Medical Students*. London: HMSO; 1957.

12 Parry N, Parry J. *The Rise of the Medical Profession*. London: Croom Helm; 1976.

13 McManus IC. Factors affecting likelihood of applicants being offered a place in medical schools in the United Kingdom in 1996 and 1997: retrospective study. *BMJ*. 1998; **317**: 1111–17.

14 British Medical Association. *Meeting the Needs of Doctors with Disabilities*. London: BMA; 1997.

15 Mellard DF, Deschler DD. LD identification: it's not simply a matter of building a better mousetrap. *Learn Disab Quart*. 2004; **27**(4): 229–42.

16 Disabilities Discrimination Act 1995. Office of Public Sector Information. www.opsi.gov.uk/acts/acts1995/ukpga_19950050_en_1

17 British Medical Association. *Career Barriers in Medicine: doctors' experiences*. London: BMA; 2004.

18 British Medical Association. *Disability Equality in the Medical Profession*. London: BMA; 2007.

19 General Medical Council. *Gateways to the Professions: advising medical schools encouraging disabled students*. London: GMC, Department of Innovation, Universities and Skills; 2008.

20 General Medical Council. *Tomorrow's Doctors*. London: GMC; 1993.

21 McManus IC. Measuring participation in UK medical schools. *BMJ*. 2004; **329**: 800–1.

22 Greenhalgh T, Seyan K, Boynton P. 'Not a university type': focus group study of social class, ethnicity and sex. *BMJ*. 2004; **328**: 1542.

23 Windeyer B. University education in the twentieth century. In: FNL Poynter, editor. *The Evolution of Medical Education in Britain*. London: Pitman Medical; 1966.

24 Attwood R. Hard work, money worries . . . and hopes for a bright future. *Times Higher Education*. 2010; **18 March**: 16–17.

CHAPTER 6

The holistic curriculum: balancing basic and psychosocial sciences with clinical practice

Barbara A Jennings and Alexia Papageorgiou

There has been a significant re-balancing of medical curricula in recent years, a process reflected in and driven by the standards first described in *Tomorrow's Doctors* in 1993.[1] The emphasis has shifted away from a curriculum dominated by fact acquisition and moved towards one that is dependent on clinical competencies and the ability to critically evaluate and apply information. The process has not been without controversy. It is viewed by some medical professionals as the erosion of the scientific knowledge base of newly qualified doctors. But by others it is welcomed because time and resources are now given to the psychosocial sciences and to communication skills. These areas emphasise professional and reflective practices and assess students according to patient-centred outcomes.

In this chapter we consider these ideas, using strands of the new medical curriculum at the University of East Anglia (UEA) as illustrations. We compare the scope of the genetics and consultation skills themes and discuss how nationally agreed standards can ensure the quality of curricula. Finally, we describe strategies to integrate these and other disciplines to produce that Holy Grail, the holistic curriculum.

BASIC SCIENCES FOR TOMORROW'S DOCTORS

The original and revised versions of *Tomorrow's Doctors* outline broad outcomes that today's undergraduate medical curriculum should achieve.[1,2,3] The emphasis is on evaluation and application of information as well as interaction with colleagues and, most importantly, patients. There is full acceptance that the acquisition of all of the knowledge, skills and attitudes that the practising doctor will need cannot be crammed into four or five years of the medical degree, and so students need to be prepared for a life-long endeavour. Modern medical educational theory proposes that students become responsible for their own learning; it encourages experiential education, for example by the use of problem-based learning (PBL); and discourages didactic teaching where factual information is presented in volume to the passive student, for example lectures to large cohorts.

The guidance given to medical schools in *Tomorrow's Doctors* may be welcome, but it is not detailed or specific for individual themes such as the sciences of genetics, anatomy and pharmacology. One message is very clear however, the amount of factual information that we insist on should only be the core minimum required for the foundation doctor to do their job after graduation from medical school.

The value of national curricula

In the fields of pharmacology and genetics there have been national initiatives to define the core undergraduate curriculum with published lists of concepts, learning outcomes and competences to prepare the foundation doctor.[4,5] These 'national curricula' serve as valuable benchmarks for comparison with the courses delivered by individual medical schools and allow for the sharing and evaluation of teaching methods and resources.

The undergraduate genetics curriculum has been developed by Peter Farndon and colleagues at the NHS National Genetics Education and Development Centre (NGEDC at http://geneticseducation.nhs.uk), after consultation with those who lead the teaching of genetics at UK medical schools. The Centre has a wider remit: to drive and co-ordinate genetics education for all UK health professionals who are working outside specialist genetic services; and the undergraduate curriculum dovetails with role-specific postgraduate curricula. This organisation was established soon after the publication of the 2003 Genetics White Paper[6] and was strongly influenced by a report commissioned by the Department of Health and the Wellcome Trust.[7] These publications identified a widening gap between the progress of genetic science and the associated knowledge of healthcare professionals. Radical changes in both the application and understanding of genetics were indicated at that time because of the emergence of a new field referred to as *genetic medicine* or *personalised medicine*, the catalyst for which was the completion of the human genome project.[8] *Genetic medicine* is much broader than the 20th century perspective on human genetics, which mainly focused on very rare diseases that were inherited according to rules first described by Gregor Mendel in 1866. This century, genetic science is touching many areas of medicine because most common diseases, and even how patients respond to medicines, are known to have a genetic component.

Traditional medical curricula led to genetics being perceived of as an overly complex, abstract science that is not of great clinical relevance because it focuses on rare diseases that most doctors would not encounter in their careers. The methods used for the delivery of genetics teaching were also failing to engage students.[5,9] This situation was clearly at odds with the enormous potential for applying genetics in medicine. Modern undergraduate medical curricula which are systems-based and integrated to consider science within a clinical context are well-equipped to address these problems. The NGEDC is also supporting individual curricula by producing electronic and other resources that encourage active engagement in tasks, such as taking family histories; and reflective patient-centred learning based on real life stories (www.geneticseducation.nhs.uk/tellingstories).

The problems with modern medical curricula

Defining a core curriculum for a given theme is a challenge; and balancing the contributions from the clinical, basic and social sciences requires flexibility and innovation. We may fully accept that it is impossible to fit expanding fields of science such as genetics into fixed time blocks, and so try to adapt a more fluid and integrated approach. But even with goodwill there are bound to be boundary disputes within faculties, which are exacerbated when academics have stronger allegiances to their own subject than to the curriculum as a whole.

There are also genuine concerns about curricula based on minimum core competencies; these include (i) an erosion of boundaries between the roles of medical graduates and other healthcare professionals, an issue also raised for postgraduate medical training;[10] (ii) the perceived lack of intellectual curiosity associated with *lighter* core science courses; and (iii) a reduction in contact teaching times for subjects like anatomy being associated with poorer exam performance.[11]

Problems will emerge, and resistance will be observed, when traditional curricula are changed; but also when new medical schools are established that follow evidence-based educational principles. One risk to be wary of is that criticism of innovations in education can lead to uncomfortable compromises, such as monitoring a student's performance by memory-based, factual examinations that are not congruent with the new curriculum design.[12]

Integration of the genetics theme within the UEA curriculum

At UEA, the genetics curriculum is delivered over the full five years of the systems-based medical degree. Each year, concepts are re-visited from a different clinical perspective but with increasing complexity. The aim of this spiral curriculum is to facilitate an increasing depth of understanding over time.[13]

TABLE 6.1 Some examples of clinical presentations associated with genetic learning outcomes in 2010

The UEA curriculum is systems-based and the clinical teaching is integrated within each PBL study week (for primary care) and within each 12 to 14 week module (for secondary care).

Year of study Systems-based module	Clinical presentation Disease	Genetic theme
Year 1 Locomotion	Abnormal gait Muscular dystrophy and Ataxia	Mendelian inheritance Mutational mechanisms Organisation of the genome
Year 2 Haematology	Haemostasis Thrombophilia and haemophilia	Mutational mechanisms X-linked inheritance Prenatal diagnosis

Year of study Systems-based module	Clinical presentation Disease	Genetic theme
Year 3 Gastroenterology	Abnormal iron indices Cancer Hereditary Haemochromatosis Family cancer syndromes	Single nucleotide polymorphisms Control of gene expression Population genetics Somatic cell genetics Penetrance and expressivity
Year 4 Paediatrics and obstetrics	The use of three- generational family history Genetic diseases	Risk assessment Laboratory tests and reports Genetic counselling Mitochondrial genetics Genomic imprinting
Year 5 Psychiatry	Family history of chronic diseases Psychosis and depression	Genotype, phenotype and environmental modifiers
Year 5 Psychiatry	Drug metabolism Adverse drug reaction	Pharmacogenetics

TABLE 6.2 Examples of genetics teaching events that integrate themes of the UEA curriculum in 2010

Teaching event	Clinical context	Faculty involved
Seminar on muscular dystrophy and ataxia	Abnormal gait and genetic disease in Locomotion module	Consultant neurologist Lecturer in molecular genetics
Workshop on genetics and the use of family history	Clinical skills session in Paediatrics module	Consultant paediatrician Clinical cytogeneticist Clinical molecular geneticist Lecturer in molecular genetics Lecturer in communication skills
Lecture on nature and nurture	Genotype, phenotype and environmental modifiers in psychiatric illness	Lecturer in health psychology Lecturer in molecular genetics

In Years 1 to 3, most of the genetics education is delivered using PBL, seminars and the occasional lecture. Core concepts are considered such as Mendelian inheritance and the organisation of the genome and molecular genetic themes are developed through the course. To give an example, in Year 1 control domains of the gene are named and in subsequent years we explain how gene expression is controlled by the interaction of response elements with proteins and other molecules. In Year 4, a theoretical understanding of inherited disease is integrated with practical skills; clinical and communication skills workshops consider the use of pedigree diagrams and genetic counselling.

The genetic themes described in Table 6.1 are introduced during PBL sessions using appropriate patient-centred, or family-centred scenarios; and so the clinical presentation acts as a vehicle to carry the core genetic concept into the curriculum. Teaching events during the week, including one day spent in a general practice, support the student's learning; and their subsequent understanding is tested and developed during PBL wrap-up sessions at the end of each week of study.

As Table 6.2 illustrates, some of the genetics teaching events require the co-operation and time of faculty members from several disciplines. This can be burdensome, because the academic and administrative workload is significant.

However, with this integrated and clinically applied approach, students engage in, and enjoy, the study of a science that has been identified by previous generations of undergraduates as an overly complex, laboratory-based discipline that is not especially relevant clinically.[5,9] Another benefit is that PBL reveals the complexity of the ethical, social and psychological issues surrounding genetics; necessitating the serious study of these disciplines too.

SOCIAL SCIENCES AND THE MEDICAL CURRICULUM

In 1974, a two-day workshop in London attempted to look at the benefits of sociology to community medicine.[14] Since then things have moved rather slowly in terms of designing, implementing and evaluating social sciences curricula in medical schools. On the positive side, the General Medical Council (GMC) which sets the standards for undergraduate medical education in the UK,[3] has outlined very clearly the need for integrating the social and behavioural sciences in the medical curricula. It emphasises that a graduate doctor should be able to apply in their medical practice both the theory and research methodologies of socio-psychological and public health sciences. In addition, the graduate doctor should be able to assimilate the GMC's ethical principles and standards and show excellent communication skills in doctor–patient–carer and inter-professional interactions.

Following the guidelines, the majority of UK medical schools have been striving to deliver an integrated medical curriculum with input from both basic sciences and social and behavioural ones for over 10 years now. As the need for input from social and behavioural sciences is relatively new in comparison to the basic sciences, the groups of academics who have been given the task to design and implement such curricula have found themselves in uncharted territories. The content, delivery and method of assessment of these subjects vary immensely from school to school and it is very common for social and behavioural scientists to operate in isolation. To overcome the isolation and the constant need to re-invent the wheel, social and behavioural scientists reached for similarly minded academics in other institutions and started a productive dialogue as to what should constitute a good enough curriculum that would meet the GMC outcomes. This pedagogic dialogue led to the development of a number of consensus statements from a number of social sciences disciplines. For example, the UK Council for Clinical Communication Skills Teaching in Undergraduate Medical Education has developed and published the UK consensus statement on the content of communication curricula.[15] The Institute of Medical Ethics (IME) has developed a model core curriculum for teaching medical ethics and law that dates back to 1998.[16] The Behavioural and Social Sciences Teaching in Medicine (BeSST) group has developed a core curriculum for psychology which is awaiting publication[17] and will continue working on other disciplines such as sociology. Health economics and anthropology are also taught in undergraduate medical schools but have not produced their consensus statements yet.

The above initiatives are indeed a very important step towards a holistic medical curriculum with the aim of producing graduate doctors who are patient-centred, competent leaders and educators as well as knowledgeable enough to cope with complex medical tasks and diagnostic uncertainties.[3]

However, current practice suggests that there is a huge gap between conceptualisation of a holistic medical curriculum and its implementation.

Using examples from the continuous effort to integrate the social and behavioural sciences into the curriculum, difficulties as well as progress will be highlighted.

Context

Nationally and internationally it is recognised by academics that Deans of medical faculties who control the allocation of resources and influence what is taught, when and by whom, may promote or hinder the integration of sciences other than biomedicine in the curriculum.[14,18]

In the UK, social sciences suffer from lack of investment in appropriately trained academics; the subjects are perceived as less important than the entrenched biomedical subjects and they usually get very little space in the undergraduate curricula where competition with basic sciences is fierce.[19] The majority of established doctors who serve as medical educators and role models of the current generations of young doctors did not get much teaching on social sciences when they were undergraduates. Their experience makes them very suspicious of the teaching of 'common sense' or 'soft topics' and their negative view gets transmitted to their students as they move through their clinical placements. On the positive side, young doctors who have experience of the teaching of social sciences, have started to slowly change the culture as they become part of the established machine.

Social scientists who are employed by UK medical schools are usually working in isolation as they do not have contact with other faculties such as sociology and psychology. Their role is usually misunderstood by their medical colleagues, they lack disciplinary support and in effect become marginalised. In addition, a number of social scientists come to a medical faculty without any previous training in medical contexts which makes it difficult for them to relate their subject to medical students, who in turn perceive such teaching as irrelevant or not important for their medical career and their exams. To overcome these barriers graduate students in social sciences must be exposed to hospital settings and community health centres in order to acquire experience of illness and its effect on the individual and society as well as interacting with doctors and healthcare professionals.[19] Finally, the involvement of clinicians in social and behavioural science teaching without any training also hinders the process of teaching, learning and assessing these subjects.

Modern medical curricula also present a huge challenge in delivering 'threads-based' social and behavioural teaching as these require a substantial administrative workload in terms of designing, delivering, evaluating and assessing such courses. In addition, the increasing number of medical students is encouraging the use of didactic lectures to large cohorts which can undermine the process of teaching and learning for these subjects. In the current financial climate, where public spending is curtailed and social scientists must focus on expanding their research profile in order to bring in valuable income, the motivation for pursuing teaching-related activities is declining. As a consequence, the much desired quality control of social sciences teaching and any progressive changes will inevitably suffer.

Content and assessment

Although the above initiatives by the UK Council for Clinical Communication, the IME and BeSST have produced useful templates for the appropriate content of social science teaching in medical curricula, it is difficult to define and translate the content into appropriate learning objectives that are directly related to medical scenarios. This is partly due to the lack of social science knowledge applicable to medicine. For example, psychologists may teach about the efficacy of psychological treatments such as CBT but they hardly ever explore the bio-behavioural process of CBT that brings about change in a patient. As Chur-Hansen *et al.* suggest, there are many psychologists with a strong research and theoretical background in biological psychology and neurosciences but they hardly ever get a teaching job in undergraduate medical education.[18] Unlike colleagues in biological sciences who have a huge amount of theory and facts to draw upon, social scientists need to modify their teaching material so that it is suitable for teaching medical students and creates a bank of knowledge for both teaching and assessment.

Although progress has been made in producing appropriate assessment methods that fit with the overall medical assessment of each medical school, it is this area along with evaluation and quality assurance of social science teaching that suffers the most at present. Given the limited administrative resources mentioned above and the lack of baseline knowledge on how to assess the social sciences in medicine accurately and efficiently, each medical school has come up with a variety of assessment methods such as:
➤ short answer questions
➤ modified essay questions
➤ multiple choice questions

➤ posters
➤ oral presentations
➤ portfolios
➤ project reports.

National bodies such as the UK Council for Clinical Communication, the IME and BeSST have all agreed mechanisms for sharing their acquired knowledge on assessment. However, there is common consensus that on many occasions these assessments do not do justice to social sciences teaching.[14]

Integration of the social sciences within the UEA curriculum

Given the above limitations of integrating social sciences within a modern medical curriculum, UEA Medical School has made substantial progress in the right direction by employing social scientists in psychology, sociology, anthropology, health economics, ethics and consultations skills. These academics have been working with the national curricula to produce an integrated and holistic medical degree. Table 6.3 below gives an example of this attempt in relation to the consultation skills thread.

TABLE 6.3 Consultation skills programme at UEA Medical School using the Calgary/Cambridge model.[20]

MB/BS	Content of teaching	Length of time	Student assessment
Year 1	Building the doctor–patient relationship, structuring the consultation, gathering information	~30 hours of experiential learning 3 hours lectures	OSCE assessment (formative and summative) Short question and answer assessment of the theory (summative)
Year 2	All of the above plus information giving	~15 hours of experiential learning 3 hours lectures	OSCE assessment (formative and summative) Short question and answer assessment of the theory (summative)

MB/BS	Content of teaching	Length of time	Student assessment
Year 3	All of the above plus shared decision making	~15 hours of experiential learning 3 hours lectures	OSCE assessment (formative and summative) Short question and answer assessment of the theory (summative)
Year 4	Special circumstances in O&G (Obstetrics & Gynaecology) and Paediatrics (e.g. taking a sexual history, breaking bad news, conveying risk)	~27 hours of experiential learning	OSCE assessment (formative and summative) Short question and answer assessment of the theory (summative)
Year 5	Special circumstances in A&E (Accident & Emergency) and Mental Health (e.g. dealing with angry patients, explaining resuscitation orders and advance directives, taking a psychiatric history, assessing mental capacity)	~30 hours of experiential learning	OSCE assessment (formative and summative)

SUMMARY

The face of medical education has changed, embracing both the challenge of ever-expanding scientific fields and the teaching of social and behavioural science within undergraduate curricula. National bodies have emerged for curricular themes such as genetics or communication skills and consensus statements about how they should be designed, delivered and assessed are in place. In order for this progressive work to continue, and for curricula to truly become integrated, the necessary resources should be put in place.

However, we are entering challenging economic times that may present barriers. In the basic science departments, progress will only continue if time devoted to teaching students is rewarded as fully as time devoted to laboratory research. Also, to firmly establish evidence-based practice, faculty support and mentoring are needed, as are protected teaching time and funding for research into the social and behavioural sciences related to medicine.

Tomorrow's doctors are expected to acquire core competencies for the various themes, and to critically evaluate, integrate and apply information, thereby encouraging a holistic approach to patient care.

ACKNOWLEDGEMENTS
Thank you to Professor Peter Farndon for useful discussions about the work of the NHS National Genetics Education Centre and to Catherine Jennings and the co-editors of this book, Penny Cavanagh, Sam Leinster and Susan Miles, for peer review and guidance.

REFERENCES
1 General Medical Council. *Tomorrow's Doctors: recommendations on undergraduate medical education*. London: GMC; 1993.

2 General Medical Council. *Tomorrow's Doctors*. London: GMC; 2003.

3 General Medical Council. *Outcomes and Standards for Undergraduate Medical Education*. London: GMC; 2009.

4 Maxwell S, Walley T. Teaching safe and effective prescribing in UK medical schools: a core curriculum for tomorrow's doctors. *Br J Clin Pharmacol*. 2003; **55**(6): 496–503.

5 Farndon PA, Bennett C. Genetics education for health professionals: strategies and outcomes from a national initiative in the United Kingdom. *J Genet Couns*. 2008; **17**(2): 161–9.

6 Department of Health. *Our Inheritance, Our Future. Realising the potential of genetics in the NHS*. Government White Paper. London: Department of Health; 2003.

7 Burton H. Addressing genetics, delivering health. *Public Health Genetics*. 2003. www.phgfoundation.org/reports/4961/

8 Collins FS, McKusick VA. Implications of the human genome project for medical science. *JAMA*. 2001; **285**(5): 540–4.

9 Telner DE, Carroll JC, Talbot Y. Genetics education in medical school: a qualitative study exploring educational experiences and needs. *Med Teach*. 2008; **30**(2): 192–8.

10 Tooke J. Aspiring to excellence. Findings and recommendations of the Independent Inquiry into Modernising Medical Careers. 2008. www.mmcinquiry.org.uk/Final_8_Jan_08_MMC_all.pdf

11 McKeown PP, Heylings DJ, Stevenson M *et al*. The impact of curricular change on medical students' knowledge of anatomy. *Med Educ*. 2003; **37**(11): 954–61.

12 Mennin SP, Kaufman A. The change process and medical education. *Med Teach*. 1989; **11**(1): 9–16.

13 Prideaux D. Integrated learning. In: JA Dent, RM Harden, editors. *A Practical Guide for Medical Teachers*. Churchill Livingstone: Elsevier; 2009. pp. 181–92.

14 Russel A, van Teijlingen E, Lambert H *et al.* Social and behavioural science education in UK medical schools: current practice and future directions. *Med Educ*. 2004; **38**: 409–17.

15 von Fragstein M, Silverman J, Cushing A *et al.* UK consensus statement on the content of communication curricula in undergraduate medical education. *Med Educ*. 2008; **42**: 1100–7.

16 Stirrat GM, Johnston C, Gillon R *et al.* Medical ethics and law for doctors of tomorrow: the 1998 Consensus Statement updated. *J Med Ethics*. 2010; **36**: 55–60.

17 Behavioural and Social Sciences Teaching in Medicine (BeSST). *Psychology Core Curriculum for Undergraduate Medical Education*. Awaiting publication. www.heacademy. ac.uk/besst

18 Chur-Hansen A, Carr JE, Bundy C *et al.* An international perspective on behavioural science education in medical schools. *J Clin Psych Med Set*. 2008; **15**: 50.

19 Larsen DE. Behavioural science in the faculty of medicine, University of Alberta. *Milbank Mem Fund Quart*. 1971; **49**(2): 219–27.

20 Kurtz S, Silverman J, Draper J. *Teaching and Learning Communication Skills in Medicine*. 2nd edn. Oxford: Radcliffe Publishing; 2005.

CHAPTER 7

Clinical teaching: past, present and future

Lesley Bowker, Christopher Hand and Richard Young

INTRODUCTION

This chapter will explore how clinical teaching has evolved and compare some of the differences in clinical teaching between primary and secondary care. We will look at how successful this teaching is in preparing our students for a career in medicine and attempt to foresee how it will need to change in the future.

A BRIEF HISTORY OF CLINICAL TEACHING
Apprenticeship

Throughout most of the 20th century, clinical teaching was synonymous with experience in hospital. Teaching was still largely based on the apprenticeship model, where a student was attached to a consultant and their team, often referred to in the UK as a *firm* or elsewhere as a *clerkship*, for a period of time (as long as three or four months). The degree of engagement often went beyond simple observation; the student undertook a social role at the bottom of a hierarchy of the medical 'family'. Students practised progressively more complex tasks until their competence almost matched that of the most junior doctor. This was a social contextual learning that could not be replicated from a book and corresponds closely to the social learning theory described by Lave and Wenger.[1]

A major advantage of this sort of teaching was that it covered the 'hidden curriculum' very comprehensively. Students emerged with a good knowledge of what was required to 'do the job' and indeed were often employed with the firms they had been attached to for their training.

Whilst many senior doctors fondly remember this style of training there were some major disadvantages. First, it was very inefficient, with students often spending hours in repetitive tasks such as routine filing of test results or phlebotomy. These roles served the firm, and were therefore socially valuable, but had little educational value. Second, the apprentice system afforded little opportunity for educationalists to influence the teaching; outmoded methods (such as teaching by humiliation) and poor role models were replicated year on year.

Clinical teaching as a part of a degree curriculum

The clearly recognisable format of undergraduate medical education, with a sharp demarcation between pre-clinical sciences and clinical training, had its origins in the early years of the 20th century. For Britain and North America at least the catalyst was Abraham Flexner,[2] who had carried out an exhaustive survey of the 155 medical schools then operating in the United States. The adoption of Flexner's ideas had considerable advantages. First, it placed scientific method, and the application of the new discoveries in physiology, pathology, microbiology and therapeutics, at the heart of the medical school curriculum. Second, it standardised the amount of basic science education which a medical student could expect to receive before encountering patients for the first time. Finally, it encouraged a level playing field for medical training with an accepted norm of five years' study.

The adoption of Flexner's reforms increased the hegemony of the 'teaching hospital' and reinforced the notion that only in such institutions could students be taught how to practise as doctors. Primary care was yet to develop into the well-resourced and organised service which it became from the 1960s onwards.

Drivers for change

By the late 20th century it was clear that the price which had been paid for such standardisation was high. The perceived relevance of basic scientific knowledge was determined by pre-clinical teachers and institutions, many of whom had little if any regular contact with clinical practice. Students complained that they were overburdened with facts about anatomy, physiology, biochemistry and so on, only to discover that perhaps only 10% of what they had learned had any routine application in clinical practice. Moreover, the delegation of such teaching to specialised pre-clinical teachers, and sometimes completely different institutions, resulted in poor integration of knowledge of basic sciences into clinical presentations. Those charged with teaching clinical medicine had themselves forgotten large parts of what they had been taught in the basic sciences.[3]

There were other disadvantages to the 'two-stage' approach to medical training. Students sometimes developed an inaccurate perception of the reality of practising medicine, based on a purely scientific education in their first two years, resulting in disillusionment for some students when first exposed to sick patients and the challenges they bring. The acquisition of important skills such as communication skills, clinical examination and intervention were confined to relatively late in the student career, and by their very nature these were recognised to be skills requiring repeated iterations to bestow both confidence and competence. Students were disadvantaged by starting the acquisition of these skills two years later than necessary. In addition, students with low aptitudes for important skills and attitudes (e.g. patient empathy) were sometimes not identified until late in the course by which time too much had been invested in their education to consider terminating their career.

Finally, there was also enormous disparity between the learning opportunities in different firms, both in terms of case-mix seen and the quality of teaching delivered. Hoffman and Donaldson investigated the constraints on teaching within the workplace and found that patient census (illness type, patient numbers, patient turnover and acuity) was the biggest single determinant of clinical teaching.[4] As curricular models have become more sophisticated the breadth of learning required dictates the type of clinical environment required for teaching.

More recently, the rise of medical education as a discipline in its own right, and the ability to point out evidence-based best practice, has accelerated the pace of change. The General Medical Council (GMC) of the UK, responsible in law for undergraduate medical education since 1858, has exerted much more pressure on curricular reform in the last few years. A competency driven culture has developed with an emphasis on teaching to valid and reliable forms of assessment such as Objective Structured Clinical Examinations rather than examining on a small selection of cases that might be encountered by junior doctors.[5]

Early pioneers in changing the way clinical experience was introduced and integrated into the undergraduate curriculum included Nottingham, Newcastle, Leicester and Southampton, most of whom were notable in being relatively new medical schools at the time that had been founded in the wake of the Todd Report.[6] At the outset these attempts to bring forward clinical experience were characterised by having a prescribed remit, such as teaching a limited range of clinical skills or 'desensitising' students to patient contact,[7] and were often confined to particular clinical settings such as primary care. These placements were intercalated within what was in effect merely a continuation of the traditional pre-clinical phase of the five-year programme. By 1994, exactly half of the academic departments of general practice in the UK provided communication skills teaching to students in Year 3 onwards, but only two departments out of 28 were involved in teaching clinical skills during the first two years.[8] Considering half of the medical profession are GPs, this imbalance needed addressing.

It would be another decade before such clinical exposure would become part of widespread attempts to provide an integrated curriculum, whereby pre-clinical sciences, clinical skills and patient management would all be taught simultaneously.[9] Whilst the adoption of integrated curricula, spurred on by the first edition of *Tomorrow's Doctors*,[10] was the main driver for change in the way clinical teaching was organised and delivered, there was a second-ary, pragmatic imperative for change. Towards the end of the 20th century it became clear that hospitals were not going to be able to provide the breadth and depth of clinical experience on which medical schools had relied for decades. Technological advances, an increasingly primary care-led health service (in the UK and North America at least) and increasing pressure to drive down the costs of healthcare have resulted in shorter episodes of patient care in hospital which are often more fragmented. The European Working Time Directive and the Calman reforms of middle grade training have both contributed to the fragmentation of the traditional medical firm.[11] Expansion of trainee numbers in the last few years has left the medical team pyramid much more broad based with relatively fewer, more hard pressed, teachers and so medical schools have turned increasingly to general practice to help provide this experience. Furthermore, there is evidence that clinical skills can be acquired as well, if not better, when taught in general practice.[12]

CLINICAL TEACHING IN PRIMARY CARE

A survey of the Quality Assurance Reports in Basic Medical Education published by the GMC,[13] in itself not a standardised or comprehensive source of information, reveals that the situation across the UK at least is complex and variable. In some medical schools clinical teaching in primary care appears to be central to the delivery of core skills and appropriate patient contacts. At the other end of the spectrum there are medical schools where primary care's role in teaching clinical skills remains as an adjunct to those functions being met in hospital clinics and wards. Utilisation of primary care for clinical curriculum delivery in some medical schools seems to reflect a desire for the specialty to 'play to its strengths' by delivering what is seen as most relevant to or best taught in that particular setting, e.g. communication skills, or case studies of families.

It is unclear why such wide variation in the place of primary care within medical school curricula persists. A very recent article commenting on this degree of variation, points out that on average only 13% of teaching is provided in primary care, and makes the case for a much more central role for the specialty in medical school curricula.[14] Possible explanations include a culture that still regards primary care as a refuge of less clinically able doctors, resource implications such as historical allocations of financial resources to teaching hospitals, and the demographics of the populations of both patients and their general practitioners in the areas immediately surrounding many teaching hospitals, which have tended to be socio-economically deprived.

The MB/BS programme of the University of East Anglia (UEA) illustrates how primary care can be utilised in the teaching of clinical skills. Whilst not held out as a template for the future, the way the course was conceived and has developed illustrates what can be achieved when starting without established structures or pre-conceptions.

The School of Health Policy and Practice of UEA successfully bid in the early years of the new millennium to offer a MB/BS degree. From the original conception of the course, primary care was seen as an integral component of curriculum delivery. The course is organised into modules each of which represents a body system, which are in turn explored through problem-based learning (PBL) presentations. The core part of each module consists of eight to 10 weeks of PBL presentations, with a new presentation for each week. This is discussed in PBL groups (10 students) at the outset of the teaching week, and the following two days or so of the teaching week then comprise lectures and seminars intended to cover the relevant pre-clinical learning outcomes. The entire fourth day of the teaching week is spent in primary care, in the same PBL groups of 10 students. The learning outcomes set for this placement are almost entirely clinical, focusing on history, examination skills, problem-solving and practical therapeutics and management. Students see patients selected by the GP tutor, based on their relevance to the particular learning outcomes of the week. The overall intention is to 'bring to life' the patients described in the scenarios used by the course, and to give students an opportunity to practise, and receive feedback on, their developing clinical skills. The week ends with a further PBL session in which students are encouraged to integrate, test and consolidate the knowledge, skills and attitudes learned during the preceding week.

The infrastructure implications of providing clinical teaching in this way are considerable. At present, the UEA Medical School has some 83 groups of 10 students being taught in approximately 53 general practices across Norfolk, Suffolk and eastern Cambridgeshire. About 110 GPs are substantially involved in the delivery of teaching, with a smaller number more peripherally involved, for example allowing students to sit in surgeries, accompanying on home visits, or supervising students' own 'mini-surgeries'. However, this tremendous effort is repaid by the satisfaction felt by the GPs and practices involved, and the fact that primary care is the most positively evaluated component of the course. In addition, the quality assurance visits of the GMC have been very favourable; for example in 2006, the visitors 'noted excellent teaching being delivered by the tutors and effective utilisation of the strengths that general practices can offer.'

CLINICAL TEACHING IN SECONDARY CARE

A fully integrated course such as that at UEA delivers clinical teaching in a more structured way with timetabled sessions throughout secondary care.

Students are rarely attached to firms and the curriculum is covered for each system's module, often by healthcare professionals from a multitude of firms and departments. For example, a student during one day of their 'nutrition' module might be timetabled to attend a structured patient teaching session delivered by a hepatologist, have a practical skills session on nasogastric feeding delivered by a specialist nutrition nurse from a different firm, and spend the afternoon observing outpatients or theatre with a surgeon.

This system requires much more central administration but benefits in being more comprehensive and almost all learning experiences are of value. Clinical educationalists have a greater opportunity to monitor and influence teaching quality and content and almost all assessment of clinical skills is done centrally rather than in the workplace.

The main disadvantage is that the teachers change so often there is little or no opportunity for social bonds to form between students and teachers. Interaction and opportunities for observation of lower ranks of junior doctor and other healthcare professionals are also limited and impersonal. Many of the teachers, who themselves were trained in a traditional model, feel this loss keenly and often complain that they see large numbers of students briefly and never 'get to know them'.

HOW WELL ARE WE DOING?

This is an obvious question to ask but a difficult one to answer. There is very little published evidence that clinical teaching is effective,[15] and yet students appear to value it. Clinical teaching can be very satisfying for both doctors and patients. However, a recent review for the GMC concluded that there were several areas where new doctors did not feel prepared for practice.[16] Insufficient ward experience was a major concern before starting the job; in particular dealing with acutely ill patients, prescribing, managing workload, performing practical procedures, and being on call. These concerns could be addressed by more clinical placements, a greater role for medical students in clinical teams, and shadowing F1 (the first year of work following graduation) jobs before starting them. Prescribing was highlighted as a weakness and ward-based teaching for this clinical skill was recommended. In summary, more experiential learning in clinical practice is needed in the undergraduate curriculum.[5] The new *Tomorrow's Doctors* has incorporated these recommendations and appears to be trying to halt, or even partially reverse, the trend away from apprenticeship learning.[13]

THE FUTURE OF CLINICAL TEACHING

There has been debate about the relevance of clinical skills in the medical practice of the future.[17] The considerable economic and political pressures, the rapid advances in technology, and the importance of lifestyle and preventive medicine threaten to marginalise the traditional role of doctors in diagnosing illness based on the application of scientific principles to an understanding of patients' symptoms and signs. However, clinical skills are as relevant, if not more relevant, than ever and the challenge of the future will be to continue to equip new doctors with these skills in spite of such pressures. Moves towards integration have made clinical skills a strand running through the entire curriculum and so for medical educators at least it would seem that the debate has already been resolved. Given that schools are now concerned with helping students acquire such skills from day one, it may be that the distinction between 'pre-clinical' and 'clinical' is an artificial one which would be better dropped.

Richard Smith, a doctor and former editor of the *British Medical Journal*, was asked to give evidence to the Royal College of Physician's working party on the future doctor.[18] He concluded that the future doctor needed at least 12 different attributes. These attributes can be grouped into three broad categories:
➤ working with patients
➤ working with professionals
➤ personal learning.

Working with patients

One thing is certain and that is the importance of learning from real patients and developing a patient-centred approach. The trend towards earlier patient contact needs to be matched by more responsibility for patients in the final two years of undergraduate training. Apprenticeship posts will help to address some of the weakness identified in training and give new doctors the confidence to know that they can do the job. However, the changes in doctors' working patterns and training will make this experience very different to what it was even 10 years ago. The pressures on clinical teaching environments outlined elsewhere in this chapter will necessitate more focused teaching using concepts like the 'one minute preceptor'.[19] This is a very simple set of steps designed to maximise the potential for useful learning in a very short interaction between learner and teacher in the clinical setting. Other contexts of care such as community hospitals, nursing and residential homes will also assume greater importance. Greater use of technology (e.g. podcasts, simulation models) will undoubtedly play a part.

The power of modern pharmacology and advances in surgical interventions have enabled doctors to heal in ways that could not have been imagined even as little as 10 years ago. But healing is more than this: comfort, reassurance and empathy are all needed when dealing with human suffering. Although these skills can be learnt, the importance of good role models will be as crucial in the future as they were in the past. Perhaps as important is the ability to help patients help themselves. Lifestyle changes and the role of preventive medicine are receiving more emphasis, but understanding the psychological processes involved and the ability to enable change should be part of the modern new doctor's repertoire.

Training in communication skills is an established part of the medical curriculum, but integrating these skills with clinical skills, clinical reasoning and ethical practice remains an underdeveloped area. Part of the problem is the complexity of the models used in communication skills training, but learning how doctors think during a consultation needs to be addressed in parallel rather than left until postgraduate education.[20]

Medical students already *learn* from patients, but in the future patients and carers will almost certainly have a greater role in teaching and assessing students.

Working with professionals

Learning to be part of a team can be learnt as well in primary care as in secondary care, as the attitudes and skills needed are common to both. Inevitably, the clinical boundaries between the health professions will change, and the value of interprofessional learning will become even more apparent. The key practical procedures that new doctors need to be able to do have been outlined by the GMC,[13] but these are not the sole province of doctors as most of these procedures are already being performed by nurses and other health professionals, and this trend is set to continue.

Personal learning
One development that will affect doctors in the future is revalidation. All doctors will have to demonstrate the quality of their clinical practice and the effectiveness of their personal learning. Advances in technology have already revolutionised access to knowledge, but recording what has been learnt and how it has been put into practice will require more sophisticated systems than we have at present. Clinical teachers will need to model reflective practice and show how experience with patients can drive learning and be incorporated into personal portfolios.

SUMMARY
The medical curriculum has changed radically over the last 40 years. The traditional pre-clinical/clinical model is being replaced by a more integrated one with early patient contact becoming the norm. More clinical teaching is taking place in primary care and this trend is likely to continue. Students need more clinical experience before becoming a doctor and this may encourage the return of the apprentice.

BIBLIOGRAPHY
Catto G. Education and training within the European Working Time Directive. *BMJ.* 2002; **325**: S69.

Dornan T. Osler, Flexner, apprenticeship and 'the new medical education'. *J Roy Soc Med.* 2005; **98**: 91–5.

Dornan T, Littlewood S, Margolis SA *et al.* How can experience in clinical and community settings contribute to early medical education? A BEME systematic review. *Med Teach.* 2006; **28**: 3–18.

Gray J, Fine B. General practitioner teaching in the community: a study of their teaching experience and interest in undergraduate teaching in the future. *Br J Gen Pract.* 1997; **47**: 623–6.

www.gmc-uk.org/about/research/research_comissioned.asp

www.gmc-uk.org/education/undergraduate/medical_school_reports.asp

www.gmc-uk.org/static/documents/content/UEA_2004.pdf

NHS Executive. *Towards a Primary Care-led NHS: an accountability framework for GP fundholding* (EL(94)72). Leeds: NHS Executive; 1994.

REFERENCES

1 Lave J, Wenger E. *Situated Learning: legitimate peripheral participation*. New York: Cambridge University Press; 1991.

2 Flexner A. *Medical Education in the United States and Canada. A report to the Carnegie Foundation for the Advancement of Teaching*. New York: Carnegie Foundation for the Advancement of Teaching; 1910.

3 Jolly B. Historical and theoretical background. In: B Jolly, L Rees, editors. *Medical Education in the Millennium*. New York: Oxford University Press; 1998.

4 Hoffman KG, Donaldson JF. Contextual tensions of the clinical environment and their influence on teaching and learning. *Med Educ*. 2004; **38**: 448–54.

5 Talbot M. Monkey see, monkey do: a critique of the competency model in graduate medical education. *Med Educ*. 2004; **38**: 587–92.

6 Royal Commission on Medical Education. *Report*. London: HMSO; 1968.

7 Cade J. An evaluation of early patient contact for medical students. *Med Educ*. 1993; **27**: 205–10.

8 Robinson LA, Spencer JA, Jones RH. Contribution of academic departments of general practice to undergraduate teaching, and their plans for curriculum development. *Br J Gen Pract*. 1994; **44**: 489–91.

9 Hastings AM, Fraser RC, McKinley RK. Student perceptions of a new integrated course in clinical methods for medical undergraduates. *Med Educ*. 2000; **34**: 101–7.

10 General Medical Council. *Tomorrow's Doctors*. London: GMC; 1993.

11 Calman K. *Hospital Doctors; training for the future. The report of the working group on specialist medical training*. London: Health Publications Unit; 1993.

12 Murray E, Jolly B, Model M. Can students learn clinical method in general practice? A randomised crossover trial based on objective structured clinical examinations. *BMJ*. 1997; **315**: 920–3.

13 General Medical Council. *Tomorrow's Doctors*. London: GMC; 2009.

14 Pearson DJ, McKinley K. Why tomorrow's doctors need primary care today. *J Royal Soc Med*. 2010; **103**: 9–13.

15 Reilly BM. Inconvenient truths about effective clinical teaching. *Lancet*. 2007; **370**: 705–11.

16 Illing J, Peile E, Morrison J *et al*. *How Prepared Are Medical Graduates to Begin Practice? A comparison of three diverse UK medical schools. Final Report for the GMC Education Committee*. London: General Medical Council/Northern Deanery; 2008.

17 Goodwin J. The importance of clinical skills. *BMJ*. 1995; **310**: 1281–2.

18 Smith R. Thoughts on future doctors. *J Royal Soc Med*. 2009; **102**: 89–91.

19 Neher JO, Gordon KC, Meyer B *et al*. A five-step 'microskills' model of clinical teaching. *J Am Board Fam Pract*. 1992; **5**: 419–24.

20 Kidd J, Patel V, Peile E *et al*. Clinical and communication skills need to be learnt side by side. *BMJ*. 2005; **330**: 374–5.

CHAPTER 8

Statistics in medical education: doctors' changing needs

Louise Swift and Gill M Price

INTRODUCTION

It is hard to believe that the use of statistical techniques in medicine really only started as recently as Bradford Hill's articles in *The Lancet* in 1937[1] and that the first undergraduate courses in medical statistics appeared only in the early 1970s. Given the novelty of the subject, advances in technology and the recent changes in the objectives of medical education, it is not surprising that the teaching of statistics at medical school has undergone enormous change in the last few decades.

The subject of statistics now appears in some form in all undergraduate medical courses in the UK. However, there is no official guidance on what should be taught or how and so medical schools differ considerably in their approach.

The UK General Medical Council (GMC) sets out the standards which undergraduate medical students must achieve by graduation in *Tomorrow's Doctors*.[2] Although it does not specify the level, amount or content of statistics teaching, this document recommends that graduates should be able to 'apply scientific method and approaches to medical research' (paragraph 12). This includes an ability to 'critically appraise . . . studies reported in the literature', 'formulate simple research questions . . . and design appropriate studies', and 'apply findings from the literature to answer questions raised by specific clinical problems'. It is interesting that the requirement in the previous edition (2003) that graduates must be able to 'analyse and use numerical data' (paragraph 26) has been dropped.[3]

Despite the GMC recommendations, research skills, including probability and statistics, are not popular subjects among undergraduate medical students. This may be because students cannot see the relevance of these subjects to their future role as a medical doctor. So do doctors really need statistics? And if so, what statistics do they need and how and when should the subject be taught?

In this chapter we look at the historical development of statistical teaching in UK medical schools concurrently with, and as a result of, changes in other related spheres. We consider some recent research on how today's doctors use statistics in their work and the value they place on statistical skills. In light of this and other research evidence we discuss the issues surrounding the teaching and learning of statistics in medical school in the future.

THE DEVELOPMENT OF STATISTICS TEACHING FOR MEDICAL STUDENTS

Several articles describe the development of statistics teaching in UK medical schools (for instance, *see* references[4,5,6]). In 1957, the GMC, in their recommendations for medical education, desired that students 'be acquainted with the principles governing the design and interpretation of clinical trials'.[7] By 1967, they were explicitly requiring teaching in 'biometric methods' and data analysis.[8] During the 1970s, most medical schools taught some statistics, usually at the pre-clinical stage, but at this time the subject was taught with a view to doing research and the emphasis was on performing calculations.

A conference of the Association for the Study of Medical Education (ASME) discussed the teaching of statistics in 1979. This precipitated a series of annual meetings for statisticians from British medical schools, currently ongoing, named the 'Burwalls meetings' after the Bristol University property at which they were first held. These meetings spawned a series of discussion papers and regular publications including some defining the aims and objectives of teaching statistics. In 1990, the journal *Statistics in*

Medicine devoted half an issue to the proceedings of the 10th anniversary meeting; this provides a good view of the issues of that time. There seems to have been dissatisfaction with traditional statistics courses presented in the early years. For example, Appleton stated that 'Courses have become too long, too detailed and irrelevant to the needs of the majority' and suggested that concepts be embedded in applied examples.[9] Clayden said that statistics teaching should be a collaboration between medical staff and statisticians.[10] Evans advocated teaching concepts as opposed to arithmetic[11] and Campbell proposed reducing the number of lectures in favour of tutorials.[12]

These developments were concurrent with, and presumably influenced by, the increased availability of computing power. Whilst acknowledging that using software enables emphasis on meaning rather than method, Murray[13] warned against its use by individuals with inadequate training. Morris reported later that at this time there was a shift away from making calculations and towards critical appraisal and interpreting statistics in the literature, even though evidence-based medicine (EBM) had not yet become widespread.[6] However, whilst courses aimed to be applied there is evidence that most were still perceived as mathematical.[9,14]

In 1991, Altman and Bland considered *why* doctors needed to know about statistics and suggested that reading and interpreting research was the main reason, along with understanding pharmaceutical company marketing material and diagnostic tests results, and doing one's own research even if only for a while.[4]

In 1993, the GMC's *Tomorrow's Doctors* instigated a major shift in the way doctors were trained. It advocated 'system-based learning' and 'self-learning' and placed less importance on the accumulation of facts.[3] This was compatible with the evolution of statistics teaching towards concepts in an applied setting.

During the 1990s, the advent of EBM increased the expectations that doctors consult and critically appraise medical research reports to inform their practice, involving a need for some statistical understanding. Electronic publishing supported by the burgeoning internet further amplified need and ability to access research literature for doctors and patients. Morris[6] suggested that any loss of identity of medical statistics in traditional form due to its integration within EBM was outweighed by the growing need for statisticians to supply the skills required to practise EBM.

In 2002, Palmer asked whether statistics teaching should be pitched at 'consumers' or 'producers' of research. He suggested that all medical students would need to become 'at least consumers of research' (p. 997) and that 21st century doctors would need sufficient critical appraisal skills to assess the internet-literature of varying quality presented by their patients.[15]

In the 2000s, as new medical schools were set up on a problem-based learning (PBL) basis the issue arose as to whether statistics teaching should be integrated within the PBL structure and, if so, how this should be done. In 2004, Bland reported that in Australia, where PBL was more developed than in the UK, no medical school had completely integrated statistics and research methods within the course. He expressed concern that if PBL were adopted more widely there would be a danger that statistics and research methods would become increasingly marginalised if not integrated into the PBL model.[16] MacDougall has also advocated that 'statistical activities are fully integrated with core material rather than bolted on', and justified this with reference to educational literature (p. 234).[17]

The issue of how, what and when statistics should be taught in an applied area is not unique to medicine. Statistics is taught at undergraduate level in most sciences and social sciences, engineering and business. Many of the changes we have seen in the teaching of medical statistics are due to the underlying evolution of statistics as a subject, namely the separation from mathematics and the availability of software allowing increased emphasis on application and interpretation. However, the adoption of EBM supported by bibliographic databases has further influenced the role of statistics in a doctor's life and invited reassessment of how an undergraduate course can best provide for this.

DO DOCTORS NEED STATISTICS? THE OPINIONS OF PRACTISING DOCTORS

Whilst the publications cited above imply that an understanding of statistics is valuable to the practising doctor, most of them were written from a medical statistician's perspective. There is little published evidence on the opinions of doctors themselves. When a sample of GPs in one region of the UK in 1997 was asked about a series of statistical terms found in medical evidence sources, between 9% and 48% of respondents said they did 'not understand the statistical term but would like to' (p. 363).[18] Windish reported in 2007 that, although resident doctors in the US showed an inadequate understanding of statistical methods, over three-quarters of those surveyed wanted to learn more.[19]

In a recent study we asked a sample of practising GPs and hospital doctors about their use of probability and statistics.[20] Almost 80% of 130 respondents considered probability and statistics important in their work. Further, about 90% of respondents considered probability and statistics useful for each of the following activities: accessing guidelines and evidence summaries, explaining levels of risk to patients, assessing marketing and advertising material, interpreting the results of a screening test, reading research publications for general interest and for non-standard treatments and, of course, for analysing numerical data.

The study also ascertained that high percentages of both GPs and consultants did indeed do each of these activities as part of their work.

The survey also asked respondents, in an open-ended question, to identify which activities in their professional life they would be able to do, or do better, if they had an improved understanding of probability and statistics. In response the doctors suggested that they would be better able to critically evaluate research and drug company literature, become more research-active, improve their clinical audit skills, better understand and be able to explain risk, and be more equipped to teach or explain things to other people (including patients, students and trainee colleagues).

These activities are compatible with the requirements of good medical practice by the GMC to keep knowledge and skills up to date; give information to patients about, for example, their condition and treatment including related uncertainties and risks; participate in audit; and exercise probity in research.[21] This should encourage today's medical students that an understanding of probability and statistics *is* relevant and useful to their future careers.

STATISTICS TEACHING: DOCTORS' OPINIONS AND TEACHERS' ASPIRATIONS

The same study asked doctors about their own undergraduate teaching.[22] Of the respondents who remembered being taught probability and statistics as an undergraduate medical student, fewer remembered the teaching as seeming useful at the time than considered it as being useful in their subsequent careers. In fact, just under half said it had *not* seemed useful at the time.[22] However, responses to open-ended questions about how their own experience of learning statistics and related subjects could have been improved, and what teaching current undergraduate students should receive, provided valuable insights into, and aspirations for, teaching statistics in medical school. The doctors' comments are reported elsewhere[22] – here we consider whether current statistical education is addressing these issues. Following the ideas embodied in the surveyed doctors' opinions and augmenting the trends outlined earlier in this chapter should provide current and future students with a more obviously relevant and more motivating learning experience.

Relevance of the teaching to future practice
Teaching of statistics, probability and quantitative research methods needs to be relevant to daily working clinical practice, including clinical decision making and explaining risk to patients. It should also enable doctors to critically review published research, the results of clinical trials, information about new treatments, evidence-based clinical guidelines and medical technology marketing material. The need for doctors to justify their decisions or recommendations to patients and peers, mentioned previously by Altman and Bland,[4] remains ever more cogent. Some students will be interested by the thought of doing research themselves, and even if this is a minority their undergraduate statistical education should give them some basic concepts and skills, enough to enable them to conduct their own research and audit with some supervision and extra study.

At the University of East Anglia (UEA), as elsewhere, we have worked on making the setting and illustrations of lectures and seminars more closely related to clinical practice. For instance, in Year 1 students do a role play explaining health risks to patients. Questions relating to a critical appraisal of a research article are often presented as hypothetical discussions with a patient. In assessed oral presentations by fourth- and fifth-year students, their self-selected case studies are presented along with a summary of their research into an aspect of the case. Suggestions from colleagues elsewhere to assist in demonstrating clinical relevance include having a senior clinical colleague give the first lecture in the series (University of Warwick) (also suggested by Evans[11]). At the University of Sheffield lectures are given jointly by a statistician and a clinician.[23] Freeman and colleagues have also tried using clinical scenario videos (for instance, of a consultation with a patient) and animations during lectures.[23]

Teaching students how to work through cases and to make decisions based on available evidence considering both risks and benefits requires sustained collaboration between statistical and clinical educators. It assumes that the clinicians are interested and conversant with EBM. Further, clinicians' own backgrounds in learning to apply statistical principles to clinical issues may hamper the extent to which they can become role models for students. Likewise, statistician-teachers need to find out more about the realities of EBM in clinical practice.

Making teaching more relevant to 'real' research should enable students to critically review published research and information about new treatments and management options, and to assess pharmaceutical literature. At UEA teaching of statistics in the MB/BS is currently aimed mainly at allowing students to interpret medical research critically, rather than to conduct statistical tests or perform calculations themselves. An issue to be addressed is the extent to which we should expect students to appraise primary medical research reports, when 'pre-digested' evidence summaries are becoming increasingly available.

It is obviously better if more recent research is used as teaching examples, and as set pieces for critical appraisal. Examples of trials currently in progress or featuring in media reports can be included. However, finding and digesting topical research for use in teaching sessions, though very rewarding and motivating, is time-consuming. Pre-digestion is often necessary since published research may use methods beyond the scope of the students' learning.

A minority of doctors need to gain skills to allow them to do their own data analysis for research or audit. Notably, the latest version of the GMC's *Tomorrow's Doctors* guidance[2] has dropped the recommendation from the previous edition[3] that students be able to 'analyse and use numerical data'. At UEA some sessions teaching the numerical analysis of data are offered in the third and fourth years but tend to be attended only by those expecting to do a quantitative research project. Students typically report that having to use the statistics they learned in the first two years of the course to design and implement a study protocol deepens their understanding and makes them more aware of the subject's relevance. Discussion is ongoing as to whether to broaden this experience to all students, while being careful not to alienate those lacking in confidence or interest, in increasing their skills in handling data.

Pedagogical issues: when and how

The teaching of statistics to medical students is often done largely in the first two years because of timetable pressure later in the course. This carries the danger that in later years, students cannot remember the meaning of, for instance, a *P*-value or a median.

There is a clear need to begin teaching statistics early and to continue building on and reinforcing earlier learning throughout the course ('spiralling'). It fits with educational models for professional learning which distinguish between understanding and the accumulation of knowledge. According to these models understanding involves cycles of applying the learning to different and more complex situations (e.g. *see* reference[24]).

Integrating statistical with clinical learning, especially where PBL methods are used for the latter, is an obvious ideal. However, it requires considerable collaboration between clinicians and statisticians, as discussed earlier. Bland reported in 2004 that although PBL teaching was more advanced in Australia than the UK, no medical school in Australia was integrating statistics within the PBL structure[16] and to our knowledge neither is any in the UK. He discussed the problems inherent in integration. These include tutors who lack confidence in statistical skills or are unwilling to use them. He makes the point that problem scenarios based on single patients are not suited to explaining most statistical methods but suggests that there is no reason why scenarios cannot be expanded beyond the patient. For instance, a patient can bring a newspaper report to the doctor. We would also add that the hierarchical nature of at least the main concepts of statistics makes it hard to weave into a set of clinical scenarios. For instance, the concept and measurement of probability is necessary in order to understand the normal or *t* distribution, which in turn is necessary to understand the assumptions and results of statistical tests. However, statistical colleagues at the University of Sheffield have developed some scenarios and are hoping to evaluate them shortly. At St Georges Hospital, probability has been integrated within communication skills scenarios.[25] Further, MacDougall in Edinburgh has developed computer-assisted learning material which integrates case scenarios with explanations of statistical concepts.[17]

Students tend to favour seminars and smaller groups, rather than lectures, for learning statistics and probability. This is supported by Bland[16] and Freeman.[23] Individual tutorials and on-demand teaching allows tailoring of teaching to students' needs, desirable in times of widening student access to medicine and consequently more varied backgrounds in numerate subjects. However, there are obvious resource implications, and this idea sadly becomes unworkable as cohort sizes continue to rise. UEA and other universities are accordingly considering the development of technological learning resources and online learning to supplement limited face-to-face contact time. Evaluation of the many different teaching media in the medical context remains to be done.

Curriculum content

Several papers have included counts of the statistical techniques used in publications (e.g. *see* references [4,26]) with a view to guiding course content. However, the popularity and need for specific techniques may change over a career and new methods will be developed. A medical education cannot prepare the student for every eventuality. It makes sense therefore that undergraduate teaching should focus on the common concepts which underlie most techniques: describing data, probability and risk, estimation including confidence intervals and testing including P-values. These fundamentals can then be applied quickly and reinforced with minimal new learning when the doctor or student needs to interpret, for instance, the results of a multiple regression within an EBM context. In this way a new statistical technique can be presented as the re-application of the initial concepts in a differing context. This is compatible with the educational idea that meaningful understanding is developed by varied application of ideas.

CONCLUSIONS

Since statistics became a subject in the medical curriculum the statistical needs of doctors have evolved both with the general trend of technology and with the changing role of the doctor. Today's doctors use and value statistical skills in their work even though many did not deem such skills relevant when first taught to them as an undergraduate. To improve this, teaching should be made more relevant to clinical decision making and to the interpretation of health research and information. However, this is time consuming and ideally requires collaboration between clinical and statistician teachers. It makes sense to teach the underlying concepts early in the medical course and then present more advanced techniques, perhaps encountered in an integrated context, as applications of these concepts. The continued reinforcement of statistical concepts from the early years by clinician-teachers later in the course maintains learning and confirms relevance.

Integration of statistics within PBL is not straightforward and requires a broadening of PBL scenarios beyond patient cases, as well as tutors who are confident with statistical ideas. The sequential nature of statistical concepts, particularly at the early stages, makes complete integration with clinical learning, via PBL methods or otherwise, difficult but ideas for such integration are being explored.

REFERENCES

 1 Hill AB. *Principles of Medical Statistics*. London: Lancet; 1937.
 2 General Medical Council. *Tomorrow's Doctors: Recommendations on undergraduate medical education*. London: GMC; 2009.
 3 General Medical Council. *Tomorrow's Doctors: Recommendations on undergraduate medical education*. London: GMC; 2003.
 4 Altman DG, Bland JM. Improving doctors' understanding of statistics. *J Royal Stat Soc Ser A*. 1991; **154**: 223–67.
 5 Campbell MJ. Statistical training for doctors in the UK. *Sixth International Conference on Teaching Statistics*. Cape Town, South Africa; 2002.
 6 Morris RW. Does EBM offer the best opportunity yet for teaching medical statistics? *Stat Med*. 2002; **21**: 969–77.
 7 General Medical Council. *Tomorrow's Doctors: Recommendations as to the medical curriculum*. London: GMC; 1957.
 8 General Medical Council. *Tomorrow's Doctors: Recommendations as to basic medical education*. London: GMC; 1967.
 9 Appleton DR. What statistics should we teach undergraduates and postgraduates? *Stat Med*. 1990; **9**: 1013–21.
10 Clayden AD. Who should teach medical statistics: when, how and where should it be taught? *Stat Med*. 1990; **9**: 1031–7.
11 Evans SJ. Statistics for medical students in the 1990s: How should we approach the future? *Stat Med*. 1990; **9**: 1069–75.
12 Campbell MJ. Response to a paper by D Clayden. *Stat Med*. 1990; **9**: 1039–41.
13 Murray GM. How should we approach the future? *Stat Med*. 1990; **9**: 1063–8.

14 Dixon RA. Medical statistics: content and objectives of a core curriculum for medical students. *Med Educ.* 1994; **28**: 59–67.

15 Palmer CR. Discussion: Teaching hypothesis tests: Time for significant change? *Stat Med.* 2002; **21**: 995–9.

16 Bland JM. Teaching statistics to medical students using problem-based learning: the Australian experience. *BMC Med Educ.* 2004; **4**: 31.

17 MacDougall M. Statistics in medicine: a risky business? *MSOR Connections.* 2008; **8**: 11–15.

18 McColl A, Smith H, White P *et al.* General practitioners' perceptions of the route to evidence-based medicine: a questionnaire survey. *BMJ.* 1998; **316**: 361–5.

19 Windish DM, Huot SJ, Green ML. Medicine residents' understanding of the biostatistics and results in the medical literature. *JAMA.* 2007; **298**: 1010–22.

20 Swift L, Miles S, Price GM *et al.* Do doctors need statistics? Doctors' use of and attitudes to probability and statistics. *Stat Med.* 2009; **28**: 1969–81.

21 General Medical Council. *Good Medical Practice.* London: GMC; 2006.

22 Miles S, Price GM, Swift L *et al.* Statistics teaching in medical school: opinions of practising doctors. *BMC Med Educ.* 2010; **10**: 75.

23 Freeman JV, Collier S, Staniforth D *et al.* Innovations in curriculum design: a multi-disciplinary approach to teaching statistics to undergraduate medical students. *BMC Med Educ.* 2008; **8**: 28.

24 Dall'Alba G, Sandberg J. Unveiling professional development: a critical review of stage models. *Rev Edu Res.* 2006; **76**: 383–412.

25 Sedgewick P, Hall A. Teaching medical students and doctors how to communicate risk. *BMJ.* 2003; **327**: 694–5.

26 Horton NJ, Switzer SS. Statistical methods in the journal. *NEJM.* 2005; **353**: 1977–9.

CHAPTER 9

Changes in medical education: examining the students' views

Susan Miles

BACKGROUND

The interest in investigating medical students' views (also referred to as collecting student feedback, conducting course evaluation, examining student attitudes/perceptions) about the environment in which they learn has increased in recent years in the face of widespread curricula change. As described in previous chapters, recommendations from the General Medical Council (GMC) in their *Tomorrow's Doctors* documents[1] have led to educational innovation ranging from small-scale changes for individual course modules to major curricula reform in all British medical schools.[2] For example, the utilisation of PBL (problem-based learning) in under-graduate medical education in comparison to traditional lecture-based courses means more small group learning, an increased need for space and other resources, and increased faculty numbers and demands on staff time. Furthermore, the shift from learning facts and repetition to a more student-centred learning approach where knowledge is understood and applied, has changed the role of teacher such that the teacher is now a facilitator of the student's learning rather than a dispenser of knowledge.[3,4,5] The teacher's role has also changed with increased use of new, particularly internet- and computer-based, learning technologies. Changes in the focus on what students are expected to learn, including integration of various elements of the curriculum and the increasing emphasis on the social sciences, has led to more diversity in the expertise of teachers. Innovative assessment methods (e.g. increased use of observed structured clinical examinations (OSCEs)) may also impact on how students experience their learning environment. The learning or *educational environment* originates from the curriculum and it includes 'everything that is happening in the medical school' (p. 9).[6] This would include, for example, values, behaviour of staff and fellow students, perceived atmosphere in learning encounters (e.g. ward-based teaching, lectures), availability and suitability of facilities (e.g. the library, computers, clinical skills resource area), how the course is organised, the hidden curriculum (what is observed and expected in clinical practice, as opposed to what is formally taught), class size, teaching skill and content of teaching material. In this chapter reasons for collecting student feedback are outlined, barriers to conducting such evaluation in the undergraduate medical education setting are highlighted, and methodological and practical issues that should be considered when setting up an evaluation system are described.

REASONS FOR EXAMINING STUDENTS' VIEWS
As medical training establishments implement changes to their curricula, so too must they examine the impact of such changes on their students' experience. Such an examination can include an assessment of knowledge/skill acquisition pre- and post-reform. But it should also consider the attitudes of medical students towards their educational environment. There are several reasons why considering student views about the educational environment in which they are learning is important. First, there is a need to evaluate the changes made to curriculum to see how well they are meeting their intended outcomes. Second, knowledge of the educational climate students are experiencing can provide information about the *quality* of the curricula.[6] As described below, there are various external requirements for educational institutes to monitor, maintain and report on the quality of the educational experience they are providing. Collecting data about student views is a valuable component of this.

Third, as described in Chapter 5, the student population on undergraduate medical courses is becoming increasingly diverse with more mature entry students, more female students, and students from different social and educational backgrounds.[7] Such diversity may well require a different course ethos to the learning environment of more historically traditional student populations in order to optimise learning and satisfaction. It is important that the educational environment is suitable for all the medical students on our courses, particularly in the face of the wide variety of teaching and assessment methods described above. Fourth, the learning environment is an important determinant of behaviour.[6] For example, evidence suggests that elements of the educational environment are related to academic achievement[8,9] and aspirations.[10] If our aim as providers of high-quality education is to produce graduates who are: 1 proficient in their areas of expertise for the next stage of their training and work, and 2 willing and able to continue to develop their knowledge/skills, then provision of an educational environment that enables this is critical.

Several authors have noted that the growing consumerism of higher education has also led to an increased interest in student views.[11,12] Expected to contribute towards their tuition fees, students are more likely to expect *value for money* from their educational experiences and may be more vocal when dissatisfied. As such, students may be more willing to provide their views about their educational environment, whether faculty wants them to or not. Consequently, incorporating a procedure for involving student feedback in the institution's standard curriculum development and quality assurance processes is likely to be of value to all stakeholders.

EXTERNAL INFLUENCES ON THE NEED TO EXAMINE STUDENT VIEWS

Harvey[11] points to two main functions of student feedback. First, it provides information that the institution can use internally to monitor curriculum quality and guide improvement. Second, it provides information that can be used externally by potential students and other stakeholders, such as accrediting or funding organisations, for quality assurance compliance. Watson[12] notes a growing emphasis on gathering student views about the quality of teaching and learning environments since the Higher Education Funding Councils were established. When created, a key role of HEFCE (Higher Education Funding Council for England) was assessing the quality of the education provided by the educational institutes it funded. At the current time, whilst the higher education institutions (HEIs) are responsible for monitoring and maintaining the quality of the education they provide, the Quality Assurance Agency for Higher Education (QAA) monitors this and reviews all HEIs, under contract from HEFCE, under the quality assurance framework. The framework includes a cyclical (6 years) institutional audit of all HEIs by the QAA and the publication of teaching quality information.[13]

The importance of student input in the quality assurance framework is apparent. QAA audit teams include student members, review teams meet with current students during audit visits, and students are able to prepare a written briefing paper for the audit which includes information about the student's experience as a learner, whether the students have a voice that is listened to, if the students know what is expected of them and the accuracy of information published by the institution.[14] Furthermore, a key component of the teaching quality information published includes information about student satisfaction, in the form of results from the National Student Survey (NSS). First conducted in 2005, the NSS is now completed by all final year students annually. It collects data about student satisfaction with various elements of their course, including teaching, assessment and feedback, academic support, organisation and management, learning resources and personal development. Data can be used by prospective students when deciding where to study, as well as providing publicly available information about the quality of education provision at HEIs.

Correspondingly, looking at medical education specifically, the GMC both sets and maintains the standards for UK undergraduate medical education. The GMC's Quality Assurance of Basic Medical Education (QABME) programme monitors the standard of educational provision.[15] This comprises two main components: the Visit Process and the Annual Return Process. For the latter, all medical schools provide a document detailing curriculum, staff or assessment changes; concerns and solutions; innovation and good practice; response to medical education issues; and progress on issues raised from QABME visits. Established medical schools are visited at least twice within a 10-year period. Similar to the QAA institutional reviews, medical students are included on the visit team and the team will meet with students during the process. Furthermore, medical schools are required to complete a questionnaire for the visit team to use as a starting point to quality assure the medical education programme, which includes a request for information about how students have influenced curriculum change. The quality assurance reports resulting from QABME visits to UK medical schools are published, giving publicly available information of the quality of the educational environment being provided.

THE CASE OF MEDICAL EDUCATION

Collecting data about medical students' views of their educational environment involves challenges not faced by many other undergraduate courses.[16] Medical students will be learning in numerous different locations, for example classrooms, hospitals (inpatient and outpatient clinics), general practice, anatomy laboratories. Much learning will take place in clinical settings where students will work with a small number of health professionals for a short period of time. In some cases, students may be learning alongside other non-teaching clinical staff who have little interest in teaching them or even in the students being there. The course is longer (normally 5 years) than most other undergraduate courses (normally 3 years). Many different teaching methods and learning opportunities will be utilised, including whole year lectures, interactive seminars, small group PBL learning, hands-on teaching and practice of clinical skills, learning through experience and observation in clinical settings.

The students will be exposed to numerous different specialists. Unlike many undergraduate courses, where specific modules are taught by a small number of subject experts (often only one teacher), medical students may have a different teacher for each session. As such, the module may have been organised by a teacher who only conducts a small number of the teaching sessions. Consequently, problems with teaching may be at the module level (in terms of structure, overall content, etc.) or the teaching session level (where different skills and styles of individual teachers may impact on student satisfaction). Commonly, medical students have less opportunity to select which modules they will undertake (with the exception of student selected studies/components). Thus, they are unable to choose to study elements they enjoy or learn with teachers they value; this may impact on satisfaction. Elements of courses may be more integrated with other teaching (e.g. pathology, sociology) rather than in subject blocks, which can have evaluation implications in terms of how to collect feedback for subject area teachers and how well topics are integrated into the curriculum as a whole. All this said, the difficulties inherent in evaluation of a medical education setting can be dealt with and overcome. In the next section, key issues that should be considered when planning to collect student views are outlined.

COLLECTING STUDENT EVALUATION DATA
Evaluation 'level'
Evaluation can be conducted at multiple 'levels', for example, at the level of the individual teacher who may provide one or more teaching sessions, the teaching session (e.g. individual lecture, PBL session, teaching ward round), module, whole course (by individual year group or by all students studying on the course), or the whole institution. The level at which the evaluation is focused will determine the type of questions to be asked. For example, when evaluating an individual teacher or teaching session, feedback might be collected on presentation skills, provision of suitable background reading, structure of session, interactiveness of session, manageable amount of material covered, etc. In contrast, evaluation at the module level might include questions about overall organisation and cohesiveness of all the teaching elements, including ordering of sessions, fitting in well with the rest of the course, availability of library and other resources, time spent on various elements of the module, appropriateness of teaching methods, etc. Evaluation at the institution level could include questions about accommodation, library and computing facilities, teaching rooms and social areas, as well as questions about learning and teaching at a more general level. Obtaining student views at multiple levels can be useful. For example, Berman[17] notes that evaluation of teachers could indicate good quality teaching – however, this would not show that the module is judged to be poorly organised with repetition of some material during the module and skimpy coverage of other material.

Evaluation method
There are numerous methods that can be used to collect data about student views of their educational environment. The method used will be determined by a number of practical issues such as the target level of evaluation, whether the goal of evaluation is summative (e.g. judging the effectiveness

of teaching for promotion purposes) or formative (e.g. identifying areas of improvement for professional development purposes), how quickly data is needed, how many students data is required from, what resources (personnel, IT) are available and the frequency of data collection. Qualitative methods, such as focus groups, are a more time consuming data collection method and may involve the input of fewer students than other methods. They can, however, provide rich data about, for example, where problems in the curriculum lie and how to resolve these. Informal methods include suggestion boxes, informal discussions with students (e.g. at the end of a teaching session) and attendance at teaching sessions. Students can provide input as representatives on module/curriculum development teams. Staff–student liaison committees are another useful way to promote evaluative dialogue between staff and students. Questionnaires/surveys are often an easy method to collect data from a large number of students. The increasing availability of computer-based forms, frequently with in-built email reminder systems, can ease the administrative burden of data collection and data entry and the convenience for responding students.

Berman[17] notes that if judgements of teaching quality rely on student views alone teachers could get good ratings through being well-liked and presenting well, but could in fact be teaching material that is out of date or set at an inappropriate level. Thus, teaching staff can also evaluate the quality of their teaching through reflection in teaching portfolios, self-evaluation of videotaped sessions of their own teaching, and expert or peer review. Likewise, when considering quality at a course or institutional level external views can form an important component (e.g. external reviews/audits by accreditation or funding authorities, external examiners' comments on perceived student weaknesses). Other methods of collecting data about the quality of the curriculum can include patient surveys and assessment of students' knowledge/skills. The evaluation of curricula outcomes can be done after graduation too by considering results of future exams, multisource feedback and surveys with graduates.

Student participation

When setting up an evaluation system a decision needs to be made as to whether participation in feedback activities will be voluntary or compulsory. Under voluntary systems evaluators need to plan how to encourage students to participate, as poor response rates lead to less valid data. Staff should be aware of the limitations inherent in the data when response rates are low, and results should be treated with caution. It is still important to consider the data, but not to be misled by it, and to take care not to act on the basis of a few extreme responses from a small number of dissatisfied students. Clearly, response rate is not an issue if participation is compulsory, but decisions need to be made as to how this will be enforced and what penalties will be imposed on students who fail to participate.

Anonymity

Students often have concerns that negative feedback they provide might be used against them by a vindictive teacher, for example through harsh marking of assessments. This can impact on how honest a student will be, which has implications for the data's usefulness. Thus, the evaluation system might be set up to allow anonymous feedback. However, with completely anonymous feedback staff are unable to come back to students if their feedback is unprofessional, if the student appears particularly stressed, or for clarification of ambiguous feedback. Thus, an intermediary can be used to collect and disseminate student feedback, acting as a buffer between the staff and students.

Designing an evaluation form

Considerable care must be taken in the design of the evaluation form. Aspects of the course on which feedback is required should be identified. Questions should not be asked for the sake of it and should only cover aspects of the course that can be changed, otherwise students' time is wasted with pointless questions. For example, if logistical issues such as room size or number of tutors dictate student group sizes then it is pointless to ask students if the group sizes are suitable. Questions should also only cover things that students can realistically evaluate. For example, it is not realistic to expect students to remember an individual lecture given 6 months ago. The inclusion of a 'not applicable' option may be useful so that students are not required to rate sessions they have not encountered, particularly when students may have had different teaching experiences at placement locations. It is also necessary to ensure that the 'hard questions' are being asked. Avoiding including questions about aspects of a course suspected of experiencing problems is unhelpful.

The right people need to be involved in the design of an evaluation form.

Successful evaluation requires faculty 'buy-in'; staff will be responsible for responding to the feedback, so it is useful to ensure that evaluation forms are covering issues that are relevant to them. This said, the concerns of curriculum developers may not be the same as those of students, so student input at the design stage is also valuable. Standardising evaluation forms is necessary if there is a need to compare feedback over time, or across different elements of the course.

Who will collect feedback, when and how?

It is important to consider the practicalities of examining student views at all stages of the evaluation process. For example, how will the data be collected and in what format: online, pen and paper or emailed template form? Related to this, how will the data be processed? Will it be entered by hand, entered using a scanner or transferred from online forms where the data is already captured?

Who will collect the data, do they have other commitments on their time and the necessary skills? Will staff collect their own feedback as part of their teaching or will it be collected centrally and come via an intermediary? To some extent this depends on the number of people involved in a course, and how their teaching is organised. For example, if a lecturer gives a block of 10 lectures in a semester it is relatively easy for them to collect their own feedback at the block's end. This is less practical where 50 lecturers give one session each in the year. Centrally administered evaluation enables course organisers to maintain more control over the process, but involves more work for a smaller number of people and consequently feedback turnaround time may be slower. However, if there is no centrally administered system then poorly performing staff may not collect their own feedback (either because they lack self-awareness about their skills or because they have no intention of changing, so do not want any feedback). If staff are collecting their own feedback, then providing a list of suitable questions that they can use as appropriate to their needs, or a standard evaluation form, is advisable so problems of poorly worded or inappropriate questions are avoided, and comparisons across teachers can be made if appropriate. Whichever system is selected, it is important that faculty recognise collection and use of feedback as integral to curriculum development, and that senior staff support the activity.

Regarding timing of data collection, it is important to check that students are actually available and not too busy to provide their feedback. For example, consider how practical it is to collect feedback when students are off-site on placement, revising for assessments, or have not actually finished the component of the course being evaluated. But student views should be provided in a timely fashion, such that they can still remember components of the course being evaluated and staff can use the data to make improvements promptly for future cohorts of students. Related to this, the frequency of data collection must be considered. It is important not to overload students with requests for feedback as they will become tired and bored, and their feedback is likely to be of less value. Likewise, it is not useful to overburden staff with data they are expected to deal with. This said, consistently collected feedback is more useful than that collected sporadically.

Closing the feedback loop

The goal of evaluation should be both to obtain data about the educational environment the students are experiencing and to *use it*. Collecting student feedback should not become a routine with no intention to actually make changes. Before collecting student feedback it is important to know who will be expected to deal with the feedback and what they should do with it. Action needs to be taken after evaluation. Such action could comprise making required improvements, further investigation to identify exactly why or where a problem exists, and consultation with stakeholders on how to remedy it.

Several authors note that it is important for feedback data to be converted into information that can be used to make change, presented back to the staff who will be expected to use it, and then both that action is taken and that students are informed about the results of their feedback.[11,12,18] This demonstrates to the students that their input has been valued. As such, it is likely to encourage future participation. Often students will not directly benefit from the feedback they have provided as it will be used to make improvements that future cohorts will experience. Without any direct evidence of change students may become disillusioned with the feedback process and refuse to participate in the future. However, if faculty report back the changes that have been made then all students will see that feedback is acted on. Requiring staff to present the results of feedback back to students will also encourage staff to actually make use of the data. However, Watson[12] notes that it is important to respond to the expectations that students have of their course and institution, rather than meeting these expectations. There may be practical or educational reasons why a particular element of the course is run the way it is; faculty need to explain this to students to indicate that their views have been considered but their expectations in this area cannot be met for the following reasons (for example, limitations on available room size for seminar teaching and small group processes working optimally when the group size is X).

SUMMARY

The current medical student is faced with a markedly different educational environment to that of even a few years ago. In the wake of extensive changes to the medical student population, teaching and assessment methods, curricula content and expectations regarding knowledge/skills to be achieved during undergraduate training, the need to examine student views of their educational environment is perhaps more important than ever. Whilst the uniqueness of the medical learning environment poses challenges for evaluation, these are far from insurmountable. Undergraduate medical training establishments need to collect student feedback to meet external requirements, and they should examine the impact of changes they implement to both ensure that the course continues to meet learners' needs and to gauge student satisfaction.

FURTHER READING

Albanese MA. Challenges in using rater judgements in medical education. *J Eval Clin Pract.* 2000; **6**(3): 305–19.

Brennan J, Williams R. *Collecting and Using Student Feedback. A guide to good practice.* York: Learning and Teaching Support Network; 2004. www.hefce.ac.uk/pubs/rdreports/2003/rd08_03/ (accessed 26.3.2010)

Kogan JR, Shea JA. Course evaluation in medical education. *Teach Teach Educ.* 2007; **23**: 251–64.

ACKNOWLEDGEMENTS

Thank you to Louise Swift for useful comments on an earlier draft.

REFERENCES

1 General Medical Council. *Tomorrow's Doctors*. London: GMC; 1993, 2003.

2 Wass V, Richard T, Cantillon P. Monitoring the medical education revolution. *BMJ*. 2003; **327**: 1362.

3 Harden RM, Crosby J. The good teacher is more than a lecturer: the twelve roles of the teacher. AMEE Guide No. 20. *Med Teach*. 2000; **22**(4): 334–47.

4 Mesko D, Bernadic M. Evaluation of the education process at the faculty of medicine. *Bratisl Lek Listy*. 2001; **102**(7): 338–42.

5 Patel VL, Yoskowitz NA, Arocha JF. Towards effective evaluation and reform in medical education: a cognitive and learning sciences perspective. *Adv Health Sci Ed*. 2009; **14**: 791–812.

6 Genn JM. Curriculum, environment, climate, quality and change in medical education: a unifying perspective. In: JM Genn, editor. *Curriculum, Environment, Climate, Quality and Change in Medical Education: a unifying perspective*. AMEE Education Guide No. 23. AMEE: Scotland; 2001. pp. 7–28.

7 Roff S, McAleer S. What is educational climate? In: JM Genn, editor. *Curriculum, Environment, Climate, Quality and Change in Medical Education: a unifying perspective*. *AMEE Education Guide No. 23*. AMEE: Scotland; 2001. pp. 3–4.

8 Pimparyon P, Roff S, McAleer S *et al*. Educational environment: student approaches to learning and academic achievement in a Thai nursing school. *Med Teach*. 2000; **22**(4): 359–64.

9 Lizzio A, Wilson K, Simons R. University students' perceptions of the learning environment and academic outcomes: implications for theory and practice. *Stud High Educ*. 2002; **27**(1): 27–52.

10 Plucker JA. The relationship between school climate conditions and student aspirations. *J Educ Res*. 1998; **91**(4): 240–6.

11 Harvey L. Student feedback. *Qual Higher Educ*. 2003; **9**(1): 3–20.

12 Watson S. Closing the feedback loop: ensuring effective action from student feedback. *Tert Educ Man*. 2003; **9**: 145–57.

13 Higher Education Funding Council for England. *Assuring Quality*. www.hefce.ac.uk/learning/qual/ (accessed 26.3.2010)

14 Quality Assurance Agency. *Handbook for Institutional Audit: England and Northern Ireland*. London: QAA; 2009. www.qaa.ac.uk/ (accessed 26.3.2010)

15 General Medical Council. *Overview of the QABME Programme*. www.gmc-uk.org/education/undergraduate/qabme_programme.asp (accessed 26.3.2010)

16 Kogan JR, Shea JA. Course evaluation in medical education. *Teach Teach Educ*. 2007; **23**: 251–64.

17 Berman E. *A Short Guide to Evaluating Teaching*. Tucson, AZ: University of Arizona; 2003. http://aer.arizona.edu/Teaching/docs/ShortGuide.pdf (accessed 26.3.2010)

18 Gibson KA, Boyle PB, Black DA *et al*. Enhancing evaluation in an undergraduate medical education programme. *Acad Med*. 2008; **83**(8): 787–93.

Index